There is beauty in everybody.
You are born with it.
It's just a matter of what you do with it,
and if you lose it,
it's like losing your soul.

—FRANCESCO SCAVULLO

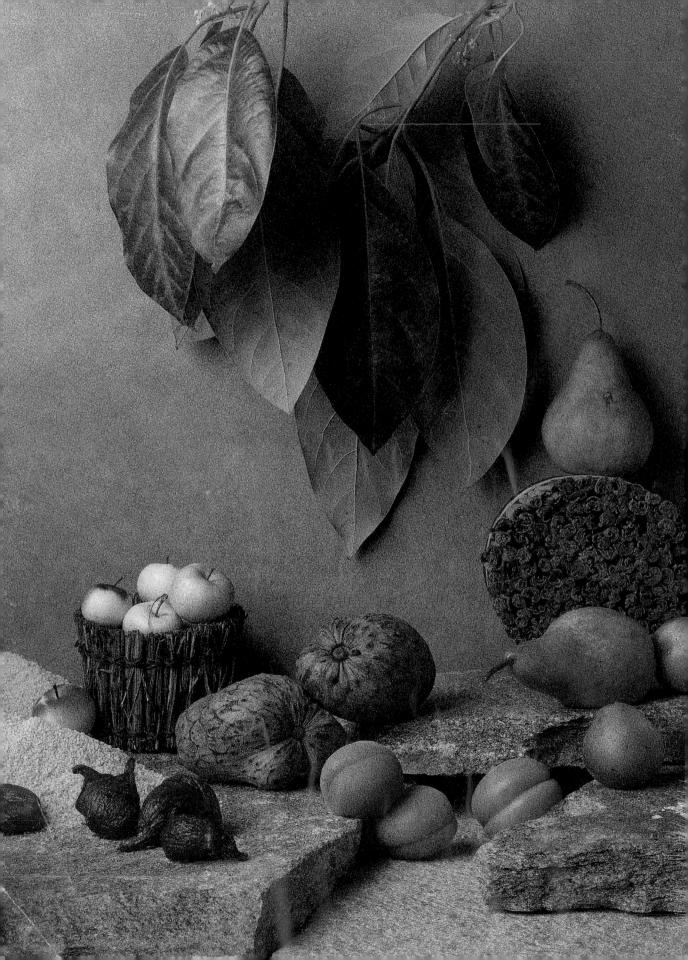

BLENDED BEAUTY

Botanical Secrets for Body & Soul

BY PHILIP B., WITH LUCY FRASER,
AND WENDY RYERSON

PHOTOGRAPHY BY
LOIS ELLEN FRANK

FOOD STYLING BY
NORMAN STEWART

TEN SPEED PRESS
Berkeley, California

TEN SPEED PRESS
P.O. Box 7123
Berkeley, CA 94707

Cover design by Nancy Austin
Cover art by Larry Kunkel
Text design by Nancy Austin and Catherine Jacobes

LIBRARY OF CONGRESS CATALOGING-IN-PUBLICATION DATA

B., Philip
    Blended beauty / by Philip B.
            p.   cm.
    Includes index.
    ISBN 0-89815-742-0
    1. Beauty, Personal. 2. Herbal cosmetics. I. Fraser, Lucy.
  II. Title.
  RA778.B13   1995
  646.7′2—dc20   95-12950
                                                      CIP

Printed in Hong Kong

FIRST PRINTING 1995

2 3 4 5 — 99 98 97 96 95

DEDICATION

To my mother, Eleanor B.
Thanks for starting me off on the right foot. I love you.

Special Acknowledgments

Blended Beauty would not have happened if not for two special people:

Wendy Ryerson, my friend and a brilliant cosmetic chemist of ten years, who burned the midnight oil countless evenings to make Philip B. products—and this book—successful.

Lucy Fraser, my friend and confidante, whose writing has guided this book through its vision. Who would have thought that an Italian encounter would result in such a lasting friendship that has progressed way beyond our love of food? I hope the ride never ends. P.S. I'm driving.

Acknowledgments

Thanks also to Diane Worthington for all your support.

Thanks to all of my friends and family who have supported my ideas and believed in me over the years.

Thanks to all of our friends and colleagues for their support and help with research, from lending professional knowledge to having their faces and heads soaked with numerous recipes: Ivan Escobell, Nancy Hildebrand, Anthony Ingrassi, Yolanda Ingrassi, Evey Kane, Martin Morgan, Ginny Read, Marina Rust, Terry Sterling, and Christopher Waite

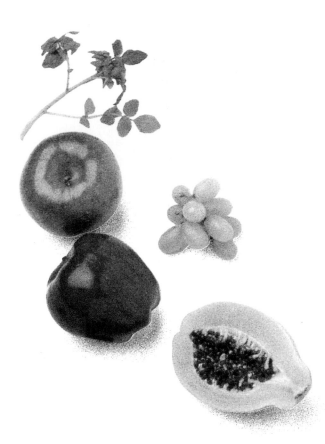

Contents

Introduction

LIFE IS ABOUT PASSION. The passion in my life has been and still is the pursuit of beauty and well being, and how we express our individuality through our inner and outer beauty. All my life, I have been fascinated with the art and science of beauty and how they constantly develop and evolve to adjust to the demands of our individual worlds. As far back as I can remember, I experimented with beauty potions, observing their effects on people visually, emotionally, and psychologically. As a small boy growing up outside of Boston, I used to join my two sisters in the kitchen, concocting homemade facial packs and body scrubs from oatmeal, flour, bran, produce, and any other feasible products we could raid from our mother's cupboards. Even back then, I would toss fruits and vegetables into the blender, just to see the end result, a cacophony of colors, aromas, and textures bursting forth, making me want to try more and more combinations.

Textures, flavors, smells, colors, everything fascinating me. My mother's perfume collection provided an abundant playground of products, which I could mix up and combine to create something more pleasing to my senses, a little off the beaten path. I remember my brother catching me in the bathroom, mixing my mother's precious perfumes, attempting to create Philip B. No. 1, and warning, "Mom's going to kill you!" But I was on a quest and nothing could stop me.

I celebrate myself and sing myself.

And what I assume you shall assume

For every atom belonging to me as good belongs to you.

—WALT WHITMAN

At the time, I didn't even realize what was transpiring. I couldn't grasp the emotional and psychological satisfaction of those experiences. I just know what I liked to smell, to taste, to feel—the heady perfumes of flowers in spring, the tangy smell of oranges pierced with cloves during the holidays, the icy brace of mint on my skin or my tongue. It was simply part of my childhood, and from adolescence onward, these natural events in my life led me on the course for which I was destined.

This kind of childhood activity would not have been possible if not for the warm, nurturing environment in which I lived. My parents had their hands full with my sisters, two brothers and, of course, me, but they always managed to give us support. We congregated in the kitchen, by far the busiest place in the house, filled with warmth and familiar smells and sounds. Eating together was important, and we gathered for dinner, prepared by my mother or by Mary, our Sicilian cook who introduced me to the wonders of Italian cuisine.

My mother instilled in me from an early age that quality was very important—the quality of raw foods as well as processed ones. She always examined labels to ensure that she was getting the best of everything. Even before organic food became popular, she tried to feed us as naturally as she could. Candy and sodas were forbidden. Fresh produce was very big. Zucchini stands out in my mind, so much so that by age ten I was convinced I had eaten my lifetime quota!

My love affair with hair began early on as well. I first started on the family cat—once I caught her, of course. I also cut my own hair all through adolescence. Cutting and shaping hair felt so natural, as though I had always done it. When I was eleven, a friend's mother, who happened to be a cosmetologist, commented on how good my own hair looked, and from that point I began to cut other people's hair. During high school, my parents encouraged me to work part-time in a hair salon on Copley Square in Boston. My perception of beauty and its place in the world began developing rapidly. I preferred the creative environment of the salon to the routines of school. Hair provided so many possibilities. Clients were like blank canvases, and I was the artist. By shaping, cutting, styling, and accenting with color, I could transform a person's looks so that every feature was maximized. The cheekbones, the jawline, every aspect of the face were all graced by new lines. I would get so turned on by accenting a woman's natural beauty, bringing out a part of her she never knew existed.

I also involved myself with chemical processing—permanent waves, highlighting, and color. I noticed immediately, however, that the chemicals took a toll on every hair they touched, depleting moisture and often leaving an artificially induced shine on the surface of the hair shaft. Somewhere in the back of my mind, I knew that there had to be a better way, a healthier way, to address the needs of hair.

I moved to Los Angeles and set up a small, intimate, boutique-style salon, a nurturing, comfortable space with cathedral ceilings, exposed wooden beams, and dried herbs and flowers gracing the walls in a wash of soft light. Through word of mouth, my clientele developed rapidly and included top Hollywood producers, actors, and studio heads.

While training with a French treatment company in the United States, I quickly realized that the percentage of active ingredients in most products was very low, promising much and delivering only a temporary remedy to dry hair and scalp. I knew that, using essential and carrier oils from nuts, plants, and flowers, I could create a treatment molecularly similar to what our bodies produce. In a corner of my salon space, I devoted myself to developing treatments using active levels of healing, pure plant extracts in combination with carrier oils. It took six months for me to develop my initial oil treatment for dry, overprocessed hair, which I eventually began using on clients. Upon completion of each treatment, custom blended every time, the results were instantaneous, and the physical and emotional reactions of my clients were tremendous. The hair would be restored to its virgin state, soft and luxurious, in 30 to 40 minutes. Without fail, every client would have the same reaction, exclaiming, "Oh my God!" Friends called me (and still do) the *alchemist*, claiming that I could create precious elements from basic beginnings.

Encouraged by the overwhelming support of my clients, the Philip B. Hair Care product line was born, launched nationwide by Neiman Marcus in 1992. With virtually no advertising except word of mouth, Philip B. Hair Care became a top producer at Neiman Marcus, praised by magazines such as *Vogue, Elle, Glamour, Mirabella, SELF,* and *W,* among others. At this point, my clientele had expanded to New York City, creating such a demand that I began leading a bi-coastal life. One week, I was immersed in the fast-paced, high-fashion, structured world of New York, the next in the sun-filled, laid-back, casual life of Los Angeles.

The Philip B. line was such a success that Neiman Marcus approached me about developing a line of body care products with active, healing properties that they would carry exclusively in the United States. In developing these new products, I used the best ingredients available worldwide, gathering the rarest and most active ingredients I could find. It was vital that these products also have aromatherapeutic properties. Aromatherapy has provided a base for all of my creations. It is an integral part of what I do. The art of aromatherapy provides neurological effects on the mind and body through the olfactory sense, or that of smell. My earliest hair and scalp treatments utilized essential oils of ylang ylang, lavender, geranium, and gardenia, combined with carrier oils such as olive and almond, to heal and restore life and luster to hair. Not only did my treatments work, but they smelled incredible, stimulating, soothing, and relaxing the senses. I learned early on in the hair business that people disliked the smell of synthetic fragrances used to mask the chemical smells prevalent in professional hair care products. With all of this in mind, I developed my product line using only natural plant extracts, up to 34% pure, which means that you aren't just getting a great fragrance, but also the natural healing properties. (The average product contains only 5% pure extract.)

While I was conducting research for these products, I traveled to Italy for a fabulous food tour with a group of American chefs and food writers. My senses came alive in this lush, beautiful country, fed by the finest of Italian cuisine. Flavors, aromas, and textures would evoke certain feelings within me, luring me deeper into the sensual experience that only certain combinations of food can bring. I call this passion—food. Like a love potion, it stirs up feelings of rapture and contentment. I was swept away by the Italian love of food and *edonista*, their lust for life, which inspired me to create food-based body care products that would nourish the exterior and awaken the senses. Everyday it smelled like I was in the middle of a garden.

Upon my return from this trip, I began consulting with a friend who is a nationally recognized chef. Based on our discoveries, I added certain food-based products to the line, signaling a departure from traditional aromatherapeutic treatments, which are based on essential oils. I wanted to take the sensory experience to new levels by utilizing ingredients never used before, modernizing the entire approach. The intensity of aroma in white truffles, carrots, green tea, and cucumber move the mind and spirit in different ways. These and other products combined together have opened my mind to new directions of sensory awareness through food. I never dreamed in all my years of research that food bases, orchestrated correctly with other components, could result in poetry for the body.

Blended Beauty brings this poetry to you at home. Using food products, some of which you may already have on your shelf and others that are easily found in your local market or health food store, you will create potions that nourish and stimulate your body and hair. The silky smoothness of one ingredient will mingle with the tingling healants of another, each taking you on its own distinctive sensory ride.

Our bodies are our gardens, to the which our wills are gardeners.

—WILLIAM SHAKESPEARE

The ingredients I use in these recipes have fed and sustained us for centuries. Certain indigenous cultures have long known of the beneficial effects that these foods have on our bodies. Our rushed, modern culture, however, has forgotten that healing can be simple and from the earth and its many gifts. *Blended Beauty* reinterprets these gifts that we consume daily and know so intimately, giving them new life and new use. Using fresh, rich avocados, tangy citrus fruits and luscious squash and melons makes the application of a beauty product so much more exciting. Blending raw foods together and applying them on hair, skin, nails, and hands takes cosmetics to a new sensory height. These new creations have inspired me so much that I may use variations of the recipes in my product line.

One of the most important things to remember while making these recipes and applying them is that you can have fun during this whole process. If you are not having fun, you are missing out on the other important component of this book. Food is serious, to be sure, but it should be a joy to work with. I suggest getting some friends together to try out the recipes. Find out which ones are right for you, what ingredients you especially like, and discover how much fun it is to get in touch with your body and your hair as you slather various mixtures on yourself. The results will reward your efforts. Your face, body, and hair will look and feel fabulous, and the experience will stimulate and renew your sensations, improving your self-esteem as well as your appreciation of everyday foods.

Using the Recipes in This Book

SELECTING RECIPES

When making a recipe that calls for produce, try to use the fresh form (i.e., fresh broccoli over frozen). If you can't find fresh vegetables and fruits, opt first for frozen and then canned. If you use canned products, make sure to use those in natural juices, never with any added sugars. Fresh produce, however, is always going to be the best.

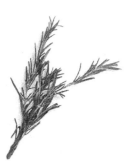

CHOOSING HERBS

If you grow your own herbs, you are in fabulous shape. Even if you don't, most markets carry fresh herbs year round. Always use fresh herbs in the recipes unless they are absolutely unavailable. Remember that herbs vary in intensity and strength, depending on where they are grown, so reduce the amount used if you notice an irritation or too potent an effect.

CLEANING AND PREPARING INGREDIENTS

Remember to thoroughly clean and wash any fresh produce. Unless they are organically grown, most fruits and vegetables have been sprayed with some kind of pesticide, and you definitely do not want any chemicals going into your skin. Also, unless the recipe calls for cooking a particular ingredient, assume that it is to be used raw, even squash and potatoes. Remove seeds as directed. Most ingredients are available in grocery stores. Some items, such as millet, may be found in health food stores. Unless directions call for a fruit or vegetable to be peeled, assume that it goes into the recipe with its skin on, thoroughly washed and cleaned.

EXTRACTS

A number of the recipes call for commercial extracts. These are concentrated versions of the original product, using water as a solvent (i.e., lemon extract is produced by squeezing the rind and mixing water with the extracted oil). Try to get extracts that are alcohol free. Since extracts are water based, they do not mix easily with oils. If a recipe contains both oils and extracts, it must be mixed or shaken before each application. These recipes are noted accordingly.

CUCUMBER EXTRACT

Several recipes call for a cucumber extract. To make ¼ cup of this extract, simply peel a whole cucumber, chop it into pieces, and blend until pureed. Strain through a paper towel or coffee filter, pressing on the pulp to extract as much liquid as possible. Discard the solids. The strained liquid is the cucumber extract.

EQUIPMENT YOU WILL NEED

The following is a list of equipment called for in the recipes:

- blender
- eyedropper
- mortar and pestle, for grinding whole spices
- cheesecloth
- string
- small whisk
- bowls (assorted sizes)
- small saucepan
- a fine-mesh strainer
- plastic cosmetic bottles
- plastic spray bottles
- resealable plastic containers with tops
- paper towels or coffee filters
- measuring cups and spoons
- cotton balls

Patch Tests

Always, always, *always* do a patch test on yourself before using any of the recipes in this book! Unlike beauty products you buy off the shelf, the ingredients in each of these recipes are often fresh and unpreserved, and consequently, more likely to be unpredictable. For instance, a very sweet papaya you buy in the summertime may have a much different chemical makeup than a semi-sweet papaya you buy in December. Therefore, each patch test you do should come from the same batch of the recipe that you're going to use, each time you make the recipe.

To do a patch test, apply a small amount of the recipe to the skin on the inside of your arm and wait twenty-four hours. If there is no reaction, it is probably safe to proceed with the treatment. If you are at all sensitive to the recipe, consult a physician or dermatologist before proceeding. Remember, you are the one responsible for making the product and you are the one responsible for your safety. Always use clean equipment and ingredients which have been thoroughly washed, and remember to discard the recipe after the time the recipe specifies to do so. If you are using eggs, be especially sure that they are fresh.

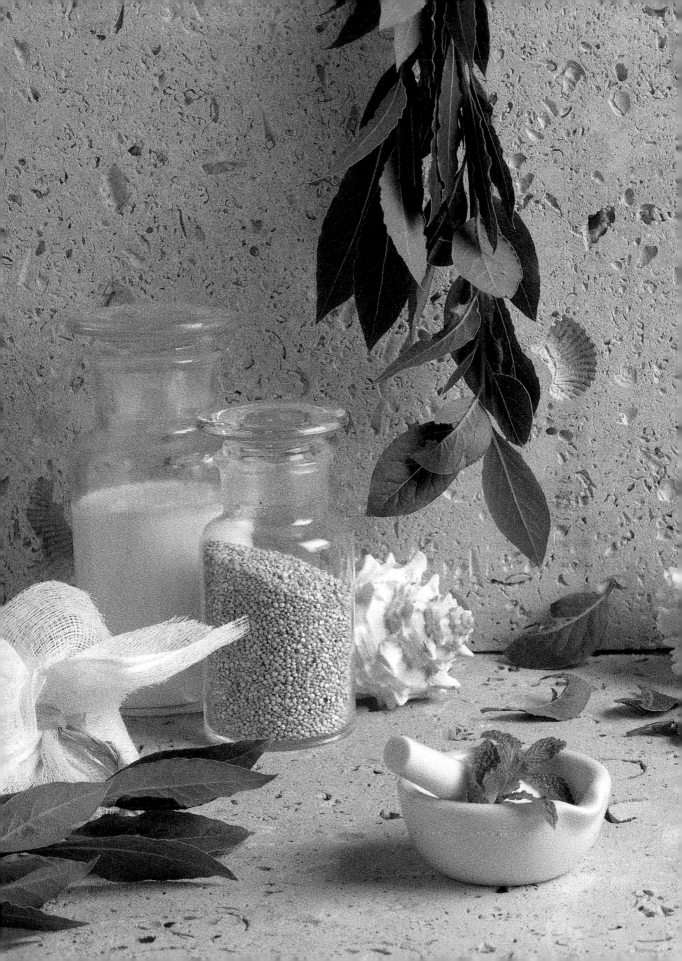

Skin & Body Care

Skin & Body Care

I N THIS CHAPTER YOU WILL FIND formulas that cleanse, exfoliate, soothe, and moisturize the skin on your body. (Formulas designed especially for facial care are given in the next chapter.) Slather on a refreshing body masque made of pureed peach and pumpkin, relax in a soothing, coconut-scented bath of moisture-rich oats and brown rice, or whirl up a cleansing body scrub containing quinoa, kale, black tea, and yogurt.

Many of the formulas in this chapter contain ingredients, such as papaya, grapes, and apples, that exfoliate the skin, or remove dead skin cells. It is important to exfoliate on a regular basis to get rid of excess layers of dry, dead cells that have built up on the skin's surface. Doing so will reveal new, healthy, glowing skin underneath. However, you should be gentle on the skin during exfoliation and body scrubs. Excessive scrubbing may result in broken capillaries in the skin. Let the ingredients used in each recipe soak in and gently do the abrasion with their own enzymes.

Beauty is not caused. It is.

—EMILY DICKINSON

Harsh weather conditions can dry out the skin, leaving it feeling rough and chapped. Bath oils and treatments are a great way to moisturize on a regular basis. I know both men and women who take a bath as part of their daily routine. It's an opportunity to relax in a warm, gentle cocoon that takes you away from your hectic world, at least for a little while, as the oils seek out and penetrate dry areas on your body. Make a bath a part of your day. The bath formulas in this chapter will relax and soothe you as they work their magic on your dry skin.

The Remedies and Special Treatments chapter contains other formulas for special types of skin and body care, including formulas designed especially for the hands and feet as well as soothing sunburn treatments.

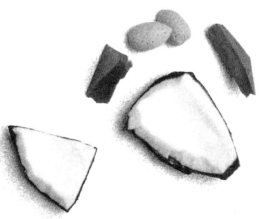

Honey-Almond Body Cleanser with Mint

For All Skin Types

Purpose: To clean and soften the skin.

Remember to do your patch test (page xiii).

mint leaves: stimulant

cucumber extract: cleanser; refresher

baking soda: cleanser; soother; softener

honey: cleanser; humectant; emollient

almond extract: emollient; scent

Mint is an incredible stimulant for the body. It sends waves of cooling, tingling pleasure through our muscles and tissues, triggering our bodies to create warming effects throughout these zones. Use fresh mint in this soap if possible; its healing properties are stronger and it smells fresher and more alive than dried mint.

This is a great cleanser for any season, although summer is a natural, as roadside stands and markets are filled with locally grown fresh herbs, such as mint, as well as natural honeys. Also, the cooling effects of the mint are wonderful relief for the skin during warmer weather.

Botanical Formula

1 cup water

2 tablespoons finely chopped mint leaves

1 tablespoon cucumber extract (see page xiii)

2 teaspoons baking soda

2 teaspoons honey (omit for oily skin)

2 teaspoons almond extract

In a saucepan, bring the water to a boil; add mint and let sit for 7 to 10 minutes. This makes a mint infusion. Let cool slightly and filter the solution, saving the liquid. To the infusion, add remaining ingredients and stir together. Apply to body or face as a liquid soap. Rinse with warm water. Follow with a cool-water rinse. Makes ¾ cup.

SHELF LIFE: Cover and refrigerate; discard after 2 days.

Honey-Orange Body Cleanser

In many cultures honey is associated with the concept of truth. Here, honey helps to reveal your true self. It cleanses and protects the skin, opening pores and drawing moisture into them. Baking soda then performs a gentle scrub cleansing, lifting away dirt, sweat, pollution, and the daily collective that builds up on the skin, restoring the purity underneath.

For Normal to Dry Skin

Purpose: To clean and condition the skin (do not use as a facial cleanser).

Remember to do your patch test (page xiii).

baking soda: cleanser; soother; softener
vegetable shortening: emollient
coconut oil: emollient; scent
orange oil: emollient; scent
honey: cleanser; humectant; emollient

Botanical Formula

1 tablespoon baking soda

¹/₈ teaspoon vegetable shortening

¹/₈ teaspoon coconut oil*

2 drops orange oil*

1 cup water

2 teaspoons honey

In a saucepan, combine all ingredients except honey and stir over low heat, bringing mixture to a simmer. Remove from heat and cool, still stirring, adding honey gradually. Product will separate; stir before using. Apply to skin (do not use on the face) as a liquid soap, gently scrubbing in a circular motion. Rinse with warm water, and follow with a cool-water rinse. Mixture may be microwaved until slightly warm before additional applications. Makes 1 cup.

SHELF LIFE: Cover and refrigerate immediately; discard after 2 days.

---

*If you cannot find oils, substitute coconut and orange extracts of each.

Milky Soft Body Cleanser

For All Skin Types

Purpose: To deep-clean, moisturize, and condition the whole body (do not use as a facial cleanser).

Remember to do your patch test (page xiii).

half-and-half: cleanser; moisturizer; A, D
potato: cleanser; toner
coconut milk: cleanser; conditioner
baking soda: cleanser; soother; softener
honey: cleanser; humectant; emollient
cucumber: astringent; toner
lemon extract: astringent; toner; exfoliant
banana extract: conditioner; scent
maple extract: conditioner; scent
skim milk: cleanser; conditioner; A, D
strawberries: cleanser; potassium
apple cider vinegar: oil remover
lemon: astringent; C

If historical accounts are correct, Cleopatra, Queen of Egypt, indulged in milk baths. Throughout the ages, women have turned to milk for skin conditioning and toning.

This cleanser, formulated for specific skin types, will leave your skin luxuriously soft and clean.

Botanical Formula

FOR NORMAL TO DRY SKIN:

2 tablespoons half-and-half
    (use heavy cream for dry skin)

$^1/_4$ potato (scrubbed, do not peel)

2 tablespoons coconut milk

1 tablespoon baking soda

2 tablespoons honey

$^1/_2$ cucumber (do not peel)

1 teaspoon lemon extract
    (omit for dry skin)

2 teaspoons banana extract
    (use 4 teaspoons for dry skin)

2 teaspoons maple extract

FOR OILY SKIN:

$^1/_4$ cup baking soda

2 tablespoons skim milk

$^1/_4$ russet potato (scrubbed, do not peel)

2 tablespoons chopped strawberries

2 teaspoons apple cider vinegar

$^1/_2$ lemon (peeled, seeded)

$^1/_2$ cucumber (do not peel)

In a blender, mix all ingredients together on medium-low speed for 45 to 60 seconds, or until smooth. Moisten skin with warm water and apply mixture, massaging it into the skin (do not use on the face). Rinse with warm water, followed by cool water. Makes $^3/_4$ cup.

SHELF LIFE: Cover and refrigerate immediately; discard after 2 days.

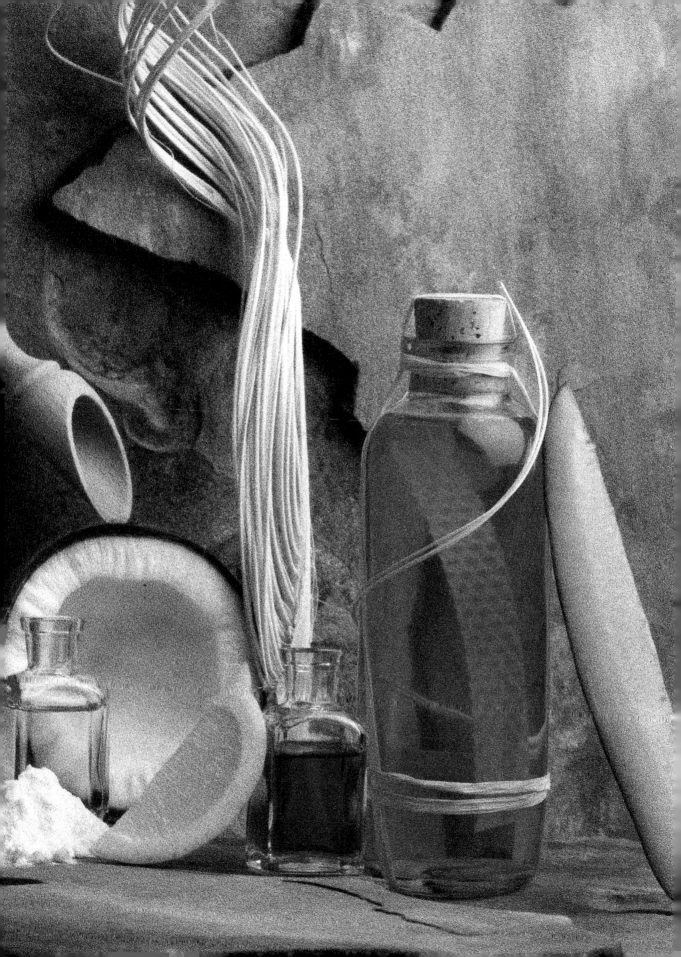

Fig–Sesame Seed Body Scrub

For All Skin Types

Purpose: To remove dead skin cells; to cleanse and moisturize new cells.

Remember to do your patch test (page xiii).

rice: toner

fig: cleanser; exfoliant

baking soda: cleanser; soother; softener

potato: cleanser; toner

egg: conditioner; toner

vegetable oil: emollient

pumpkin: moisturizer; **A**

avocado: moisturizer; **A, C, D, E;** potassium; thiamin; riboflavin

half-and-half: cleanser, moisturizer; **A, D**

almonds: exfoliant

sesame seeds: exfoliant

lemon juice: astringent; **C**

Emperor Augustus of ancient Rome had a penchant for fresh figs. So much, in fact, that he tended to the palace fig trees himself, cultivating and nurturing the exotic, rich fruit. My own love affair with figs began with a trip to Italy, where, during a lunch in the countryside, I feasted on fresh figs with prosciutto. The sweet flesh caressed my palate, leaving me intoxicated.

The cleansing power of figs is renowned and their enzymes also help exfoliate old skin layers. Here, figs are combined with almonds and sesame seeds for a vigorous, tingling body scrub. After dead skin cells have been lifted away, avocado, milk, and pumpkin condition, moisturize, and soften the skin, leaving your body invigorated and smelling as delicious as it feels.

Fresh figs are available for only a few months—June through October—so plan to indulge in this scrub when they are in season. For the rest of the year, you could simply leave the fig out.

Botanical Formula

1 cup long-grained rice

1 cup warm water

1 fresh fig

3 tablespoons baking soda

1/8 russet potato (scrubbed, do not peel)

1 whole egg

2 teaspoons vegetable oil

1 cup chopped pumpkin flesh

1/8 avocado (peeled)

2 tablespoons half-and-half

1 cup ground almonds

1 cup sesame seeds

FOR DRY SKIN:

Omit the russet potato

Use heavy cream instead of half-and-half

FOR OILY SKIN:

Omit egg and vegetable oil

Use skim milk instead of half-and-half

Add 2 teaspoons lemon juice

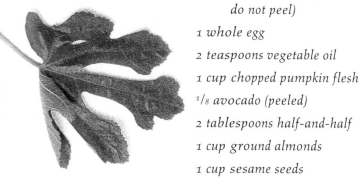

Soak rice in water for 30 minutes. Strain, saving liquid and discarding the rice. In a blender, mix the rice water with all other ingredients except almonds and sesame seeds on medium-low speed for 45 seconds. Add almonds and sesame seeds and blend for another 45 seconds to disperse. Moisten the skin with warm water, then apply the scrub in a circular, massaging motion. Scrub gently, as the exfoliants can damage the skin if applied too roughly. Rinse with warm water and follow with cool water. Makes 3 cups.

SHELF LIFE: Cover and refrigerate; discard after 2 days.

Equatorial Enzyme Pack

These formulas are designed to provide exfoliation of dead skin cells for either sensitive or nonsensitive skin. In the formula for nonsensitive skin, a papaya, source of the enzyme papain, aggressively goes after dead skin cells, while the avocado and oatmeal moisturize and protect the new skin underneath.

The sensitive skin formula uses grapes, a milder exfoliant that, along with the pineapple, also protects skin against irritation and inflammation. Both of these formulas will reveal new, fresh skin that looks and feels smooth and silky.

NOTE: Apple seeds contain toxins—be sure to core your apple.

Botanical Formula

FOR NONSENSITIVE SKIN:

1 cup quick rolled oats

1 cup warm water

1 papaya (peeled, seeded)

1 apple (cored, do not peel)

1/4 grapefruit (peeled, seeded)

2 tablespoons pineapple flesh

1/2 avocado (peeled)

1/2 lemon (peeled, seeded)

FOR SENSITIVE SKIN:

1 cup quick rolled oats

1 cup warm water

1/4 cup pineapple flesh

10 white seedless grapes

1/4 apple (cored, do not peel)

1/2 cucumber (do not peel)

1 tablespoon almond extract

1/2 russet potato (do not peel)

2 egg whites

In a small bowl, mix the oats with the water and let the mixture sit for 15 minutes to allow the oats to absorb the water. In a blender, combine all ingredients except for the oatmeal mixture. Blend on medium-low speed for 45 seconds, or until smooth. Add oatmeal to mixture, blending on medium speed for 20 to 30 seconds. When thoroughly blended, apply to the skin and leave on for 20 to 30 minutes. Wash off with a gentle cleanser or soap. Makes 2³/₄ cups.

SHELF LIFE: Cover and refrigerate immediately; discard after 2 days.

For Normal or Sensitive Skin

Purpose: To remove dead skin cells and blemishes on the body.

Remember to do your patch test (page xiii).

oats: cleanser; soother; B, E
papaya: exfoliant; conditioner; papain; A, C
apple: exfoliant; malic acid; A, C
grapefruit: exfoliant; cleanser; C
pineapple: anti-inflammatory; exfoliant; A,C; bromelain
avocado: softener; A, C, D, E; potassium; thiamin; riboflavin
lemon: astringent; C
grapes: exfoliant; anti-inflammatory
cucumber: astringent; toner; exfoliant
almond extract: emollient; scent
potato: cleanser; toner
egg whites: ingredient binder

Indian Summer Body Pack

For All Skin Types

Purpose: To gently moisturize sensitive, stressed, or chapped skin.

Remember to do your patch test (page xiii).

sweet potatoes: moisturizer; A, C

broccoli: moisturizer; A, C; riboflavin; calcium; iron

macadamia nut oil: moisturizer

spaghetti squash: moisturizer; emollient; A, C; iron

corn: toner; A

cucumber extract: toner

egg whites: ingredient binder

This recipe draws upon the natural healing effects of fall harvest. Spaghetti squash provides an emollient, leaving a smooth finish on the surface of the skin. Combined with the broccoli and sweet potatoes, the squash completes an effective moisturizing and conditioning team, rehydrating and smoothing the skin. This marvelous trio will give skin back its familiar glow and softness. This special body spread will treat your skin, leaving it with new elasticity and silky smoothness.

Botanical Formula

$^1/_2$ cup cut-up dark-skinned sweet potatoes (uncooked, peeled)

$^1/_2$ cup cut-up broccoli (stems and florets)

1 tablespoon macadamia nut oil (omit for oily skin)

$^1/_2$ cup cut-up spaghetti squash (raw flesh, no seeds)

1 cup canned corn (with liquid)

5 tablespoons cucumber extract (see page xiii)

2 egg whites

In a blender, mix all of the ingredients together on high speed for 45 seconds, then on medium speed for another 45 seconds. When mixture is thoroughly blended, gently pat it on the skin and let it sit for 15 to 20 minutes. Rinse off with warm water. For best results, apply to skin twice a week. Makes 2 cups.

SHELF LIFE: Cover and refrigerate immediately; discard after 2 days.

Quinoa-Kale Cleansing Scrub and Body Polish

Quinoa makes the perfect centerpiece for a cleansing scrub. This ancient Peruvian grain rolls gently over the skin, exfoliating and lifting dead skin cells without damaging the texture or integrity of the skin. Quinoa has a deliciously nutty aroma and is packed with all essential amino acids, which are present in the skin. Fresh from your garden or market, tender sweet peas and crunchy kale give the skin a blast of vitamin A, which increases the rate of cell growth. The fragrances of orange and almond light up this fabulously creamy, grainy-textured scrub. Your skin will be revitalized and tingling and will be free of flat, lackluster old skin cells.

For All Skin Types

Purpose: To exfoliate, clean, smoothe, and condition skin.

Remember to do your patch test (page xiii).

black tea: anti-inflammatory
baking soda: cleanser; softener; soother
kale: softener; A, C; folic acid; calcium; iron
peas: emollient; A, C
almond extract: emollient; scent
orange extract: emollient; scent
yogurt: conditioner; cleanser
millet: exfoliant
quinoa: exfoliant; essential amino acids; E, B

Botanical Formula

1 black tea bag

$1/4$ cup boiling water

2 tablespoons baking soda

$1/2$ cup chopped kale

$1/2$ cup cooked peas

$1/4$ teaspoon almond extract

$1/4$ teaspoon orange extract

$1^1/2$ cups yogurt (use nonfat yogurt for oily skin)

1 cup millet

$1^1/4$ cups quinoa

Steep tea bag in $1/4$ cup boiling water. Let cool slightly. In a blender, mix hot tea with baking soda, kale, peas, and extracts on medium speed for 30 seconds, or until smooth. Bits of kale will remain throughout mixture. Add yogurt, millet, and quinoa and blend mixture on medium speed for 2 to 4 minutes, depending on the power of your blender. Mixture should be grainy but smooth. Moisten skin with warm water. Apply mixture liberally to the skin in a circular, massaging motion. Leave on for 5 minutes. Rinse off with warm water. Follow with a moisturizer. Makes $3^1/2$ cups.

SHELF LIFE: Cover and refrigerate immediately; discard after 2 days.

Pumpkin Power
Deep Moisturizing Body Oil

For Normal to Dry Skin

Purpose: To provide an intensive, overnight moisturizing treatment for skin.

Remember to do your patch test (page xiii).

pumpkin: moisturizer; **A**
coconut oil: softener
olive oil: softener
corn oil: softener
peanut oil: softener
cucumber extract: refresher

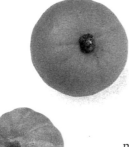

Every fall my family would drive through New England, taking in the glories of the autumn foliage. We would always stop at one of the roadside stands and buy several pumpkins, heavy and cumbersome and filled with rich, dark, sticky flesh.

That rich, fragrant flesh can also provide moisture for your skin. This moisturizer is ideal for nighttime use because it is so oil rich. Slather it on as liberally as you like, massaging it deeply into your pores. You'll wake up in the morning feeling like a newborn baby.

Botanical Formula

$^1/_2$ cup chopped pumpkin flesh

2 tablespoons coconut oil*

2 tablespoons olive oil

2 tablespoons corn oil

2 tablespoons peanut oil

2 tablespoons cucumber extract (see page xiii)

In a blender, mix all ingredients on medium-high speed for 1 minute. Apply to the skin with a circular massaging motion. Wrap extra-dry areas with plastic for extra effect. This can be used nightly. The cucumber extract may separate, so whip by hand for subsequent applications. Makes $1^1/_8$ cups.

SHELF LIFE: Cover and refrigerate; discard after 2 days.

---

*If coconut oil is not available, substitute walnut oil.

Amaretto Body Silk

The almond, one of our favorite nuts, gives a wonderful richness to the tantalizing elixir amaretto, a liqueur made from almonds. Originally cultivated in India, the sweet, exotic aroma of the almond fills the air, giving us heady thoughts of warm, sultry nights in foreign lands. Incorporate these wonderful elements into an oil-rich moisture base and you have a sensational soothing elixir for the body.

Coconut extract adds some softening, as well as a tropical scent. Slipping on this daily body treat will result in soft, silky skin. It's the perfect weapon against the drying effects of winter.

Botanical Formula

1 teaspoon macadamia nut oil

1 teaspoon olive oil

1 teaspoon canola oil

1 teaspoon corn oil

1 teaspoon coconut extract

1 teaspoon almond extract

Mix all ingredients together in a cosmetic bottle. Apply by massaging into the skin. This can be used daily. Mix well before each application. Makes 2 tablespoons.

SHELF LIFE: Store in a cosmetic bottle; do not refrigerate; discard after 1 week.

For Normal to Dry Skin

Purpose: To condition the skin's surface by increasing the water content of the top layer of the skin.

Remember to do your patch test (page xiii).

macadamia nut oil: conditioner
olive oil: conditioner
canola oil: conditioner
corn oil: conditioner
coconut extract: softener
almond extract: softener

Laurel Bay Mint Bath

For All Skin Types

Purpose: To soothe, cleanse, and refresh the body and to relieve stiff, aching joints.

Remember to do your patch test (page xiii).

mint: stimulant; refresher
bay leaves: healant
coconut oil: conditioner
**almond extract: anti-
   irritant; softener**
lemon juice: oil remover; C

Greek mythology includes a story of the god Apollo, who is known for wearing a laurel bay wreath upon his divine locks. He wears the wreath in honor of Daphne, a beautiful nymph he pursued in an amorous chase. At Daphne's bidding during the chase, her father turned her into a laurel bay tree to protect her. Daphne's beauty is honored in this bath as bay leaves target stiff and swollen joints and reduce inflammation.

This bath draws upon very simple and subtle qualities of invigorating mint and soothing bay leaves that, when combined, take us to new sensory depths. In one luxuriously intoxicating soak, the body is healed, soothed, stimulated, and moisturized.

Botanical Formula

1 cup chopped fresh mint

1 cup chopped bay leaves

1 teaspoon coconut oil*

1 teaspoon almond extract

FOR OILY SKIN:

Omit coconut oil and almond extract

Add 1 teaspoon lemon juice

In a mixing bowl, toss all ingredients together. Place mixture into a 12-inch by 12-inch cheesecloth square; tie into a pouch with string. Submerge pouch in bath with hot water running. Water should be quite hot in order for herbs to infuse properly. After the water is a comfortable temperature, slip in and bathe for at least ¹/₂ hour. Makes enough for 1 bath.

SHELF LIFE: Discard after 1 use.

---

*If coconut oil is not available, use coconut extract.

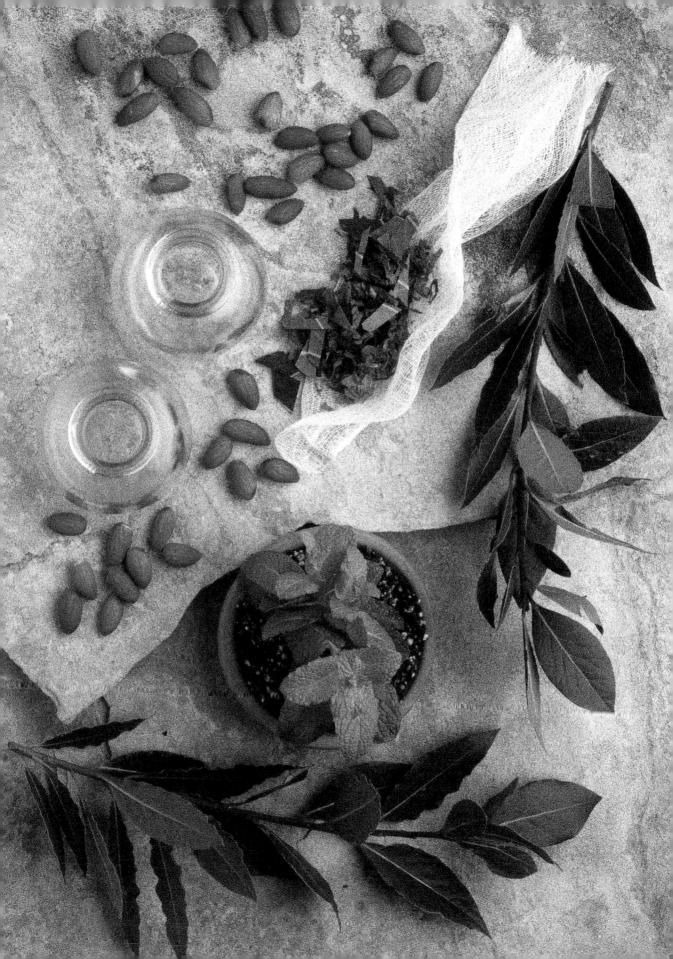

Three-Bean Body Salad
Skin-Conditioning Body Masque

Although beans have been cultivated for at least 6000 to 7000 years, many early varieties began to vanish during the 20th century. Luckily for us, a revival of "heirloom" bean cultivation by small farmers is resulting in the re-emergence of older, often more interesting varieties.

Rich conditioning from beans combined with other treasures from the garden gives new beauty and life to your body as you spread on this smooth, creamy moisturizing masque. It's especially useful for extra-dry areas of the body, such as elbows and upper arms. Your skin will feel renewed, moisturized, and conditioned and will glow with a new softness and silky texture.

Botanical Formula

$3/_4$ cup water

2 tablespoons chopped parsley

2 tablespoons vegetable shortening

$^1/_2$ cup cooked soybeans

$^1/_2$ cup cooked garbanzo beans or chick-peas

$^1/_2$ cup cooked lima beans

$^1/_2$ avocado* (pitted, peeled)

$^1/_4$ cup pine nuts

3 large white mushrooms

$^1/_4$ cup chopped collard greens

FOR OILY SKIN:

Omit avocado, pine nuts, and vegetable shortening

Add 1 tablespoon lemon juice

Bring water and parsley to a boil, then simmer for 15 minutes, creating an infusion. Remove from heat and let cool slightly. In a separate saucepan, heat vegetable shortening slowly until liquefied. Remove from heat. If using dry beans, soak overnight and then simmer until soft. Combine beans, avocado, pine nuts, shortening, mushrooms, collard greens, and parsley infusion in a blender and mix on medium speed for 2 to 4 minutes, or until smooth. Mixture will spread more easily when warm. Apply to body by gently patting onto skin, pressing firmly to ensure adhesion. Leave on for 10 minutes at the most. For future uses, let mixture reach room temperature and reblend with $^1/_2$ cup water if necessary in order to make mixture spreadable. Makes 2 cups.

SHELF LIFE: Cover and refrigerate; discard after 3 days.

---

*Avocado will turn a dark greenish brown color when exposed to air; this does not affect the product.

Peach-Pumpkin Smoothie Conditioning Body Masque

"Peaches and cream" is a term frequently used to describe beautiful, healthy, glowing skin—skin that is rosy, soft, and supple, much like a ripe peach. Unfortunately, not everyone has peaches-and-cream skin. This formula combines ingredients that remove excess oil from the skin while it restores a balance of moisture all over the body and improves the complexion. Skin will be soft and glow with the warm rosiness of health.

For All Skin Types

Purpose: To condition, tone, and moisturize skin.

Remember to do your patch test (page xiii).

Botanical Formula

2 teaspoons honey

2 tablespoons half-and-half

¹/₂ peach (with skin)

¹/₂ cup chopped pumpkin flesh

¹/₈ teaspoon instant coffee

1 tablespoon cucumber extract (see page xiii)

2 egg whites

FOR OILY SKIN:

Add 1 tablespoon lemon juice

Use skim milk instead of half-and-half

FOR DRY SKIN:

Use 3 tablespoons honey

Add 1 tablespoon each banana and coconut extracts

Use heavy cream instead of half-and-half

honey: conditioner; emollient
half-and-half: conditioner; A, D
peach: conditioner; A, C
pumpkin: moisturizer; A
coffee: anti-inflammatory
cucumber extract: astringent
egg whites: ingredient binder
lemon juice: oil remover; C
banana and coconut extracts: softener; conditioner

In a blender, mix all ingredients together on medium-low speed for 45 seconds, or until smooth and slightly whipped. Apply to the skin with a steady spreading motion; leave on for 15 to 20 minutes. Rinse with warm water. Makes 1¹/₂ cups.

SHELF LIFE: Cover and refrigerate immediately; discard after 2 days.

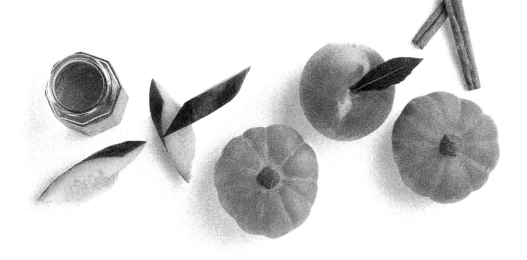

Aromatic Fruit Salsa Masque for Face and Body

For All Skin Types

Purpose: To exfoliate, tone, soften, and condition skin.

Remember to do your patch test (page xiii).

pineapple: exfoliant; anti-inflammatory; **A, C;** bromelain

mango: softener; **A, C, D**

honeydew melon: softener; **C**

cantaloupe: softener; **A, C**

banana: softener; potassium; **C**

pear: soother

kiwi: emollient; **C**

peach: softener; **A, C**

grapes: anti-inflammatory

cilantro: aromatic stimulant

pectin: ingredient binder; toner

watermelon: astringent; **A, C**

This refreshing fruit salsa masque blends readily available fruits for a tingling, cooling body treat that exfoliates, softens, and moisturizes the skin. Salsa is becoming such a staple in our eating experience; make this one part of your regular beauty diet. The combination of fruits, from rich, fragrant mangoes to crisp, refreshing melons, is so gentle that you can use this every day. Its cool, soft texture feels great going on and, after you rinse it away, dead skin cells are gone, replaced by rosy skin that glows with the beauty of the season.

Botanical Formula

2 tablespoons chopped pineapple flesh

1 mango (peeled, pitted, and chopped)

$^1/_2$ cup chopped honeydew melon

$^1/_2$ cup chopped cantaloupe

$^1/_2$ banana or plantain (peeled)

$^1/_4$ pear

1 whole kiwi (peeled)

$^1/_4$ peach

10 seedless grapes

$^1/_2$ cup cilantro (coriander leaf)

1 pack liquid pectin

FOR OILY SKIN:

Omit cantaloupe

Add $^1/_2$ cup watermelon

In a blender, mix all ingredients together on medium speed for 2 to 4 minutes, or until thoroughly mixed. Mixture will be slightly lumpy, but consistent. Place in a bowl and let sit in the refrigerator for at least 30 minutes. This gives the pectin a chance to gel. When mixture is slightly gelatinized, apply liberally to skin. Let sit for 20 to 30 minutes. Rinse off with warm water. Makes 2$^3/_4$ cups, enough for 1 application.

SHELF LIFE: Refrigerate if not used immediately; discard after 2 days.

Orange-Coconut Body Moisturizer

This fabulously rich and smooth daily moisturizer is designed especially for mature skin. Obtaining moisture in the skin is essential because our bodies produce less oil as they mature.

This formula goes on smoothly without feeling oily or sticky. Light touches of coconut and orange oil will embrace your skin, giving a sexy silkiness. If you prefer other scents, try extracts of strawberry, chocolate, and vanilla for a "Neapolitan" sensation. Delicious!

For Mature Skin

Purpose: To moisturize, rehydrate, and soften older skin.

Remember to do your patch test (page xiii).

Botanical Formula

1 teaspoon rice bran oil

1 teaspoon avocado oil

1 teaspoon canola oil

1 teaspoon walnut oil

2 teaspoons lemon juice

2 teaspoons lime juice

$^1/_2$ teaspoon coconut oil*

$^1/_4$ teaspoon orange oil*

rice bran oil: moisturizer
avocado oil: moisturizer
canola oil: moisturizer
walnut oil: moisturizer
lemon juice: astringent; C
lime juice: astringent; C
coconut oil: emollient; scent
orange oil: emollient; scent

In a small saucepan, heat all ingredients together; let cool and pour into a cosmetic bottle. Apply by rubbing into skin, all over. Lemon and lime juices will separate from the oils. For future uses, shake to mix oils and juices and apply as usual. If using scented extracts, shake to mix with oils also, as extracts are water based. Makes 2 tablespoons.

SHELF LIFE: Store at room temperature; discard after 1 week.

___

*If coconut and orange oils are unavailable, use extracts. If you desire a stronger scent, use more of each extract.

Black Tea Body Masque with Almond and Peppermint

For All Skin Types

Purpose: To smooth the skin and give it a silky finish.

Remember to do your patch test (page xiii).

black tea: soother; astringent

sage leaves: stimulant; healant

thyme leaves: stimulant; antiseptic

gelatin: thickener

honey: humectant

almond extract: emollient

peppermint extract: emollient

Just feeling this thick, amber-toned masque in your hand will give you an idea of how it embraces and penetrates the skin. The gelatin helps the masque bind beautifully to your body, holding in the conditioning powers of the tea and honey.

A relaxing warmth will spread over you as the herbs heal the body and stimulate the senses. After you've rinsed the masque away, your body will feel refreshed and toned, with a smoother, tighter appearance. The extracts will leave a soft, rich aroma on your skin with a silky, warm finish.

Botanical Formula

$1^1/_4$ cups water

2 black tea bags

1 tablespoon chopped sage leaves

1 tablespoon thyme leaves

$^1/_2$ packet unflavored gelatin

$^1/_2$ teaspoon honey

$^1/_4$ teaspoon almond extract

$^1/_2$ teaspoon peppermint extract

Bring the water to a boil in a saucepan; immerse the tea bags, sage, and thyme in it, reduce heat, and simmer for 25 minutes; remove from heat and cool slightly. Stir in gelatin, honey, and extracts. Let sit in refrigerator for 8 to 12 hours or until firm (it should have a gelatinous consistency). Apply to the body, smoothing mixture evenly over skin. Leave on for 15 minutes, then rinse with warm water. Makes 1 cup. For entire body, double the recipe.

SHELF LIFE: Cover and refrigerate; discard after 5 days.

Hearts of Palm Firming Masque for Neck, Body, and Face

This masque contains a combination of richly textured softeners, conditioners, and toners that smell and feel great on the skin. Toners such as hearts of palm and celery are great on older skin.

The longer this masque is left on, the more it will tone and condition. The deep, penetrating action firms and smoothes all over. It's great on the neck and throat, areas where skin feels less firm as it matures. Try it on your face and the rest of your body as well, especially around the knees and upper arms. Your body will feel invigorated and refreshed, with a silky, soft texture and tone.

Botanical Formula

$^1/_2$ *cup chopped hearts of palm*

$^1/_4$ *cup wheat germ*

$^1/_4$ *cup powdered milk*

2 bay leaves

1 stalk celery

$^1/_4$ *russet potato (scrubbed, do not peel)*

1 teaspoon mint

$^1/_2$ *cucumber (do not peel)*

1 teaspoon vanilla extract

1 teaspoon coconut extract

2 egg whites

In a blender, mix all ingredients together on medium-low speed for 45 seconds, or until pureed. Using your fingers, rub onto the skin with a gentle circular motion. Be extra gentle on neck and throat area. Let sit for 15 to 25 minutes, then rinse well with warm water. Use 2 or 3 times a week. Makes 1 cup.

SHELF LIFE. Cover and refrigerate immediately; discard after 3 days.

For Mature Skin

Purpose: To tighten and tone skin, leaving it looking more youthful.

Remember to do your patch test (page xiii).

hearts of palm: conditioner; toner
wheat germ: conditioner; E
powdered milk: softener; toner; A, D
bay leaves: healant
celery: toner
potato: toner; astringent
mint: stimulant
cucumber: refresher
vanilla extract: emollient; scent
coconut extract: emollient; scent
egg whites: ingredient binder

Oatmeal, Rice, and Coconut Bath

For All Skin Types

Purpose: To soften, smooth, and rehydrate rough, dry, tired skin.

Remember to do your patch test (page xiii).

oats: conditioner; **B, E**

brown rice: toner; fiber; **B, E**; calcium; iron

coconut extract: softener; scent

black tea: healant; soother

powdered milk: cleanser; emollient; **A, D**

Rice is considered one of the great food staples of the world. This ancient grain, cultivated for over 5000 years, feeds not only half of the world's population, but now the skin as well.

A bath is the perfect environment for the nourishing qualities of rice. The rice in this bath mixture will tighten and tone your skin, restoring elasticity, while the black tea soothes your aching joints and muscles and the scent of coconut rises amidst the steam. You deserve this right now, so slither in and enjoy.

Botanical Formula

1 cup oats

1 cup brown rice

1 teaspoon coconut extract

5 black tea bags (emptied) or 2 tablespoons loose tea

1 cup powdered milk

Mix all ingredients in a mixing bowl. Divide mixture in half, storing one half in a covered container for future use. Place the other half of the mixture into an 8-inch by 8-inch cheesecloth square; tie into a pouch with a string. Run a bath with very hot water and submerge the pouch in the water. Squeeze the pouch a few times to fully hydrate the ingredients. When water has cooled to a comfortable temperature, slip into bath. Pouch may remain in bath. Try to stay in the bath for at least 30 minutes for full benefit. Makes 3 cups, enough for 2 baths.

SHELF LIFE: Discard after 1 use.

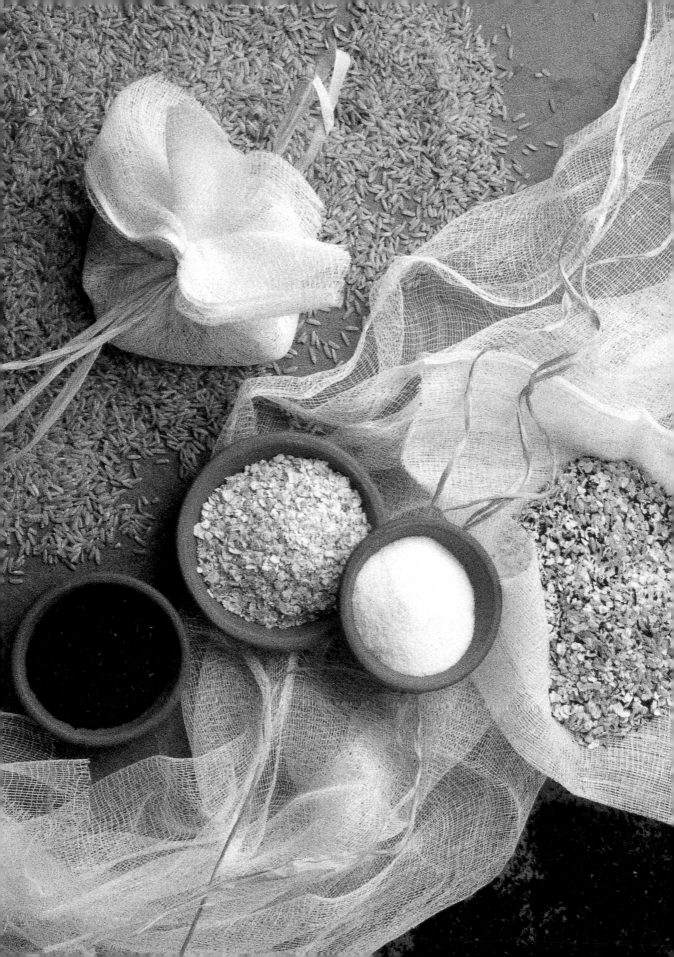

Rosemary–Wheat Germ Body Toner

For Mature Skin

Purpose: To tone mature skin, tighten and smooth existing wrinkles, and deter new wrinkles.

Remember to do your patch test (page xiii).

sage leaves: antiseptic

rosemary leaves: antiseptic; stimulant

wheat germ: nutrient; moisturizer; E

cucumber: astringent; refresher

potato: toner

alfalfa sprouts: toner; astringent; protein; C

lemon extract: refresher

Wheat germ is full of vitamin E, which is excellent for any type of skin, but especially for more mature skin, which lacks the elasticity and tone associated with youth. Vitamin E is believed to retard the aging process in skin, as well as help heal scars and redness.

The combination of wheat germ and toners in this formula will help diminish the appearance of wrinkles and retard the development of new wrinkles. Your skin will be noticeably softer and more supple, feel cleaner and look better.

Botanical Formula

$1/2$ cup water

2 tablespoons chopped sage leaves

2 tablespoons chopped rosemary leaves

$1/4$ cup wheat germ*

$1/2$ cucumber (do not peel)

$1/4$ russet potato

1 tablespoon alfalfa sprouts

1 teaspoon lemon extract

Bring water, sage, and rosemary to a light boil; reduce heat and simmer infusion for $1/2$ hour. Let cool and, in a blender, mix infusion with remaining ingredients together on medium speed for 1 minute, or until pureed. Filter solution through a paper towel or coffee filter, discarding solids. Put liquid into a small cosmetic bottle and apply to face, gently wiping with a cotton ball. Let toner absorb into skin and follow with a moisturizer. Use daily. Makes 1 cup.

SHELF LIFE: Cover and refrigerate; discard after 3 or 4 days.

---

*Wheat germ turns rancid quickly due to its high oil content, so I recommend keeping it in the refrigerator.

Honey-Banana Milk Bath

The banana tree, which is actually a very large herbaceous plant, leads a short but extraordinary life. Growing to full size in a little over a year, it produces one bunch or "hand" of bananas and then dies. The hand ranges from about 50 to 300 bananas or more, depending on the variety and size of the plant.

Bananas are wonderful humectants, helping to draw moisture into the skin. This moisture-rich bath treatment is also filled with other wonderful conditioners and emollients, such as milk, which cleanses and also evens out skin tone. Your skin will be left smelling like sweet bananas and feeling soft and supple.

For All Skin Types

Purpose: To cleanse, soften, and soothe the entire body.

Remember to do your patch test (page xiii).

milk: conditioner; A, D
banana: moisturizer; potassium; C
honey: moisturizer
baking soda: cleanser
eggs: conditioner
coconut milk: conditioner

Botanical Formula

1 cup milk

1 whole banana (peeled) or 1 tablespoon banana extract*

$^1/_4$ cup honey

1 tablespoon baking soda

2 whole eggs

$^1/_2$ cup coconut milk

In a blender, mix all ingredients together on medium-low speed for 30 seconds. Add to bath while water is running. Remain in bath for at least 30 minutes. Makes 2 cups, enough for 1 or more baths.

SHELF LIFE: Cover and refrigerate; discard after 2 days.

---

*The extract will not be quite as effective as a real banana, but it does clean up easier. Banana may be mashed by hand and placed in a cheesecloth bag to avoid having banana flesh in water.

Orange-Coconut Bath Oil

For Normal to Dry Skin

Purpose: To deeply condition skin in a bath environment.

Remember to do your patch test (page xiii).

macadamia nut oil: conditioner
rice bran oil: conditioner
canola oil: conditioner
olive oil: conditioner
avocado oil: conditioner
orange oil: scent
coconut oil: scent

A number of my clients have asked me about overall body moisturizing. Most commercial products don't really moisturize or even hold in the moisture that your body already has. They simply give the illusion of soft skin. This formula is different: Most of the oils used are occlusive, so as they bind to the skin, they retain moisture and softness. After using this bath oil, the scents of coconut and orange will cling gently to your skin, and your body will feel soft, warm, and protected.

Botanical Formula

1 tablespoon macadamia nut oil

1 teaspoon rice bran oil

1 tablespoon canola oil

1 tablespoon olive oil

1 teaspoon avocado oil

1 teaspoon orange oil*

$^1/_4$ teaspoon coconut oil*

In a small saucepan, slowly heat all ingredients until warm. Stir frequently, making sure ingredients are homogeneous. The coconut oil will need to dissolve thoroughly. Remove from heat and pour into running bath water, right under the faucet. The oils will not mix with the water. They will, however, bind to the skin's surface during bathing. For best results, use twice a week. Makes 4 tablespoons, enough for 1 bath.

NOTE: If the sides of your bathtub become oily after the bath, use a rinse of apple juice or apple cider vinegar to clean them.

---

*If orange oil and coconut oil are not available, use extracts.

Orange-Coconut Deodorant

Start every morning with this fresh-smelling, effective alternative to the commercial products you've probably been using your whole life. First apply the blended liquid—a mixture of greens, vinegar, and orange and coconut extracts. When dry, follow it with the simple powder of baking soda and cornstarch to absorb wetness and provide a smooth finish over the deodorant solution. It's a natural, healthy way to stay dry.

Botanical Formula

LIQUID:	POWDER:
2 tablespoons chopped iceberg lettuce	¹/₄ cup baking soda
2 tablespoons chopped fresh parsley	¹/₄ cup cornstarch
2 tablespoons chopped watercress	
1 teaspoon apple cider vinegar	
3 drops orange extract*	
2 teaspoons coconut extract*	

In a blender, mix the botanical ingredients together on medium-low speed until liquefied. Strain mixture through a paper towel, saving the liquid, which is the deodorant. Sift powder ingredients together in a bowl. Apply the liquid under the arms with a cotton ball. After solution dries, apply powder to underarms to absorb perspiration and wetness. Makes 2 tablespoons.

SHELF LIFE: Cover and refrigerate immediately; discard after 2 days.

---

*Amounts of orange and coconut extracts may be increased to cover aroma of vinegar.

For All Skin Types

Purpose: To gently scent the body naturally.

Remember to do your patch test (page xiii).

iceberg lettuce: astringent; soother
fresh parsley: anti-irritant; A, C
watercress: astringent
apple cider vinegar: astringent
orange extract: scent
coconut extract: scent
baking soda: desiccant
cornstarch: desiccant

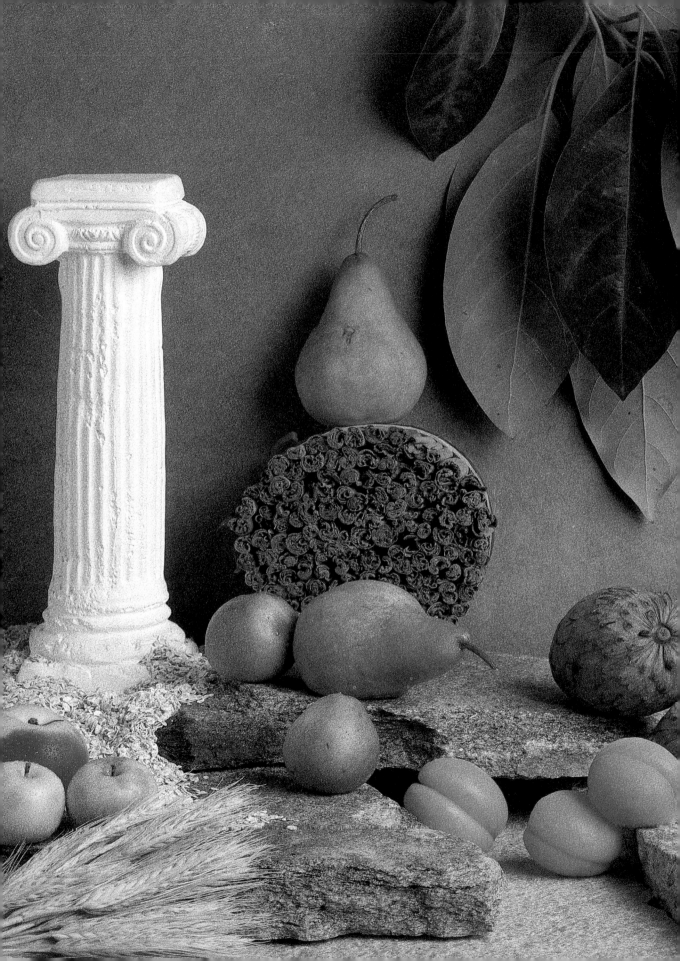

Facial Care

Facial Care

THE SKIN ON YOUR FACE, especially around the eyes, is delicate and deserves the best care you can give it. Use the formulas in this chapter to cleanse, tone, exfoliate, and moisturize your face naturally. Try a tropical frappé made of pineapple, banana, apple, and almonds to gently cleanse and exfoliate your face. Make a citrus-scented toning masque of honey and avocado. Or create a facial mist containing tea and lime extract for a quick pick-me-up during the day.

Those with sensitive skin or mature skin, as well as those who suffer from acne, will find here facial formulas created especially for their needs. The Honey-Oatmeal Facial Masque and the Whipped Oatmeal–Sesame Seed Scrub Cream are formulated especially for sensitive skin. If you've avoided exfoliating for fear of causing irritation in your skin, try one of these recipes. If you have mature skin, it is important to exfoliate the dead skin that collects around wrinkles and makes them more noticeable. Try the Apple-Pear Nighttime Wrinkle Lotion for gentle exfoliation. The body also produces less oil as it ages, meaning that older skin needs constant replenishment of the skin's lost moisture. The Coco Palm Facial Moisturizer is designed for just this purpose. And if you have acne, the Watercress-Papaya Acne Cleanser and the Apple-Grapefruit Acne Masque will bring deep-cleaning relief.

All of my formulas use only the freshest and purest ingredients. Most of the oils in the moisturizing formulas, such as canola oil, sesame oil, and olive oil, are occlusive, which means that they form an effective seal on the surface of your skin, retaining moisture and softness. These oils truly rehydrate and protect your skin, rather than simply giving it a fleeting feeling of softness that soon is gone.

The facial toners are useful for all skin types. Their purpose is to remove any excess oil or dirt that cleansing might have missed and any residual traces of the cleanser itself. A toner should leave your skin feeling refreshed and tightened without drying the skin or depleting vital moisture. Some of the toners in this chapter are designed especially for oily skin; in these I've boosted the astringent and oil-removing ingredients to remove oily buildup and to tighten pores, giving the face a smoother, cleaner look.

> *Nature gives you the face you have when you are twenty. Life shapes the face you have at thirty. But it is up to you to earn the face you have at fifty.*
>
> —COCO CHANEL

Creamy Cucumber Facial Cleanser

Purpose: To cleanse the entire face without drying.

Remember to do your patch test (page xiii).

cucumber: cleanser; refresher
potato: toner
baking soda: cleanser
egg: ingredient binder; toner
yogurt: cleanser; conditioner; lactic acid
lemon juice: oil remover; C

The cool, refreshing quality of cucumber provides instant relief to skin. This is a great daily wash that can be used on the entire body as well as the face. Its fresh, wholesome smell and smooth, creamy texture will bring your skin to life, whether it's first thing in the morning or late at night.

Botanical Formula

1/4 cucumber (chopped, do not peel)

$^1/_8$ russet potato (chopped, do not peel)

1 teaspoon baking soda

1 whole egg

$^1/_4$ cup plain yogurt

FOR OILY SKIN:

Use nonfat yogurt

Add 2 teaspoons lemon juice

Increase baking soda to 2 tablespoons

Use egg white only; discard yolk

In a blender, mix cucumber and potato together on medium speed for 20 seconds. Add remaining ingredients and blend on low speed for 1 minute. Moisten face with warm water and apply cleanser with a washcloth in a gentle circular motion. Rinse clean with warm water; follow with cool-water rinse. Makes 1^1/$_2$ cups.

SHELF LIFE: Cover and refrigerate; discard after 2 days.

Apple-Pear Nighttime Wrinkle Lotion

Dead skin cells build up on the surface of your skin, making wrinkles more pronounced. These cells need to be peeled away gently, especially if you have mature skin. By using only the juices of the apple, lemon, and lime, and not the flesh of each, this formula results in an exfoliation process that is gentler on mature skin, yet still effective. Removing these dead cells produce a cleaner, smoother appearance to your face.

Botanical Formula

1 teaspoon apple juice

1 teaspoon lemon juice

1 teaspoon lime juice

2 tablespoons buttermilk

1 tablespoon rosemary leaves

3 seedless grapes

$1/_4$ pear

2 egg whites

Blend all ingredients together on medium speed for 30 seconds. Using a cotton ball, dab mixture on areas around the eyes and wherever wrinkles have developed. Let dry, then rinse with warm water. Use no more than 3 times a week. Follow with a moisturizer. Makes 1 cup.

SHELF LIFE: Cover and refrigerate immediately; discard after 4 days.

For Mature Skin

Purpose: To reduce the appearance of wrinkles and mildly exfoliate the dead cells congregating around the wrinkles on face.

Remember to do your patch test (page xiii).

apple juice: exfoliant
lemon juice: exfoliant; C
lime juice: exfoliant; C
buttermilk: moisturizer; exfoliant; lactic acid
rosemary leaves: antiseptic; refresher
grapes: anti-inflammatory; A, C
pear: soother
egg whites: toner

Fragrant Facial Moisturizers

For All Skin Types

Purpose: To hold moisture in the skin and maintain soft and pliable appearance of skin.

Remember to do your patch test (page xiii).

light sesame oil: moisturizer
coconut oil: moisturizer
orange extract: emollient
banana extract: emollient
vanilla extract: emollient
lemon extract: emollient; astringent
lime extract: emollient; astringent
olive oil: moisturizer
rice bran oil: moisturizer
macadamia nut oil: moisturizer

It is imperative to provide moisture to the skin (even oily skin needs to be softened and conditioned). These moisturizers have been formulated for specific skin types. Intensive oils that help hold in the moisture are used in the dry skin formula. Just a few drops applied to the face will pamper and protect your skin. In the formula for normal skin, sesame and coconut oil are balanced by extracts which reduce excess greasiness from the oil, causing them to penetrate quickly. Citrus extracts are great for the oily skin formula. They give an astringent tightness to skin, making pores seem smaller.

Botanical Formula

FOR NORMAL SKIN:

1 teaspoon light sesame oil

¹/₄ teaspoon coconut oil

1 teaspoon orange extract

1 teaspoon banana extract

1 teaspoon vanilla extract

FOR DRY SKIN:

1 teaspoon olive oil

¹/₄ teaspoon coconut oil

1 teaspoon rice bran oil

1 teaspoon light sesame oil

1 teaspoon macadamia nut oil

2 teaspoons lemon extract

FOR OILY SKIN:

1 teaspoon lemon extract

1 teaspoon orange extract

1 teaspoon lime extract

DIRECTIONS FOR DRY SKIN: Over low heat, warm ingredients, mixing together until coconut oil is liquefied. Transfer to a small plastic container. Using a dropper, put 3 drops of mixture onto a fingertip, and gently apply to facial area with a dabbing action. Mixture may be microwaved until slightly warmed for future uses. Makes ¹/₈ to ¹/₄ cup.

DIRECTIONS FOR NORMAL SKIN: Follow directions for dry skin formula. Extracts will separate slightly from oils, so whisk together before using. Makes 1¹/₂ tablespoons.

DIRECTIONS FOR OILY SKIN: In a small cosmetic bottle, combine ingredients, shaking vigorously. Follow application for dry skin, using less of formula on t-zone. Makes 1 tablespoon.

SHELF LIFE: Store at room temperature; discard after 1 week.

Tropical Facial Frappé

In the 19th century, pineapples were considered an exotic rarity. Families would bring out a pineapple only for very special visitors, thus establishing it as a symbol of hospitality. Pineapples are much more plentiful today, but still valued for their luscious, juicy flesh, full of tangy, sweet flavors that linger long after the fruit is eaten. The gentle acid plays with our palate, tempting us to eat more. It is that very quality that makes it perfect for a facial scrub.

Pineapple is a naturally gentle exfoliant and, more importantly, an anti-inflammatory. Bromelin, the enzyme it contains, digests protein, quickly and effectively breaking down dead skin layers. The ground almonds in this facial scrub cleanse the skin, penetrating pores and lifting away dead skin cells that the fruit enzymes have begun digesting, creating a smoother texture on the face. The dry flakiness that existed before will be gone, leaving a new layer of gorgeous, glowing skin fed on some of the best of the tropics.

NOTE: Apple seeds contain toxins—be sure to core your apple.

For Nonsensitive Skin

Purpose: To remove dead skin cells from the skin's surface with a scrub.

Remember to do your patch test (page xiii).

pineapple: exfoliant; anti-inflammatory; A, C; bromelain
apple: exfoliant; malic acid; A, C
almonds: cleanser; exfoliant
lemon juice: astringent; C
lime juice: astringent; C
banana: moisturizer; potassium; C
almond extract: conditioner
gelatin: fortifier

Botanical Formula

$^1/_2$ cup chopped pineapple flesh

1 whole apple (cored and chopped, do not peel)

$^1/_4$ cup finely ground almonds

1 tablespoon lemon juice

1 tablespoon lime juice

$^1/_2$ banana

1 teaspoon almond extract

$^1/_2$ packet unflavored gelatin

In a blender, mix all ingredients except gelatin on medium speed for 20 seconds. Add gelatin and blend for another 20 seconds. Let mixture sit for at least 10 minutes to allow gelatin to set slightly. Apply evenly to the entire face and neck area. Leave on for 15 to 20 minutes, then rinse with warm water. May be used twice a week as needed. Makes 1 cup.

SHELF LIFE: Cover and refrigerate; discard after 2 days.

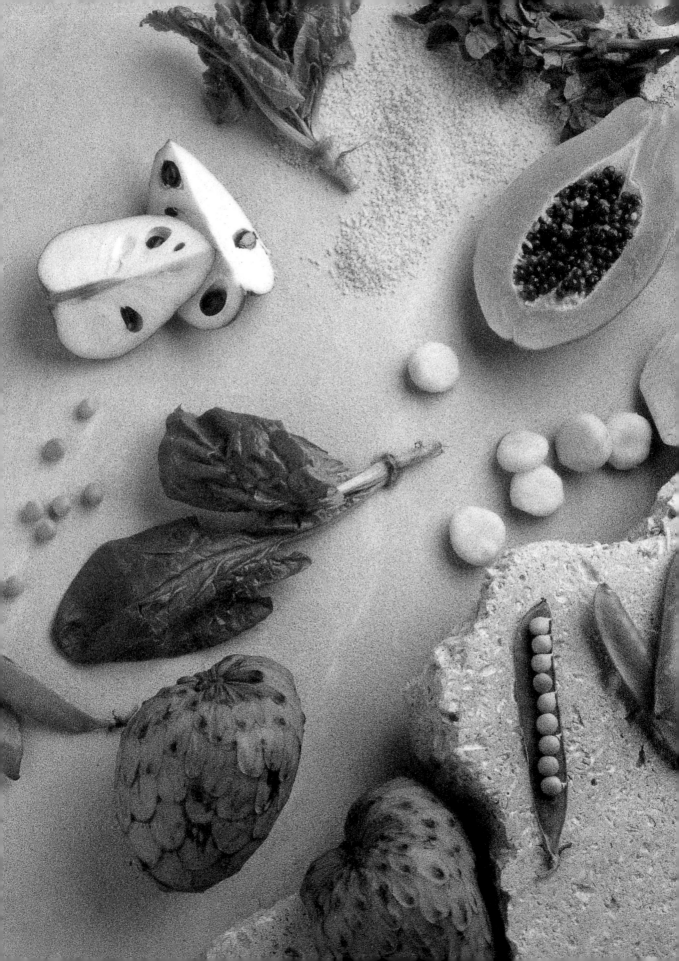

Cherimoya-Couscous Moisturizing Facial Scrub

This is truly a global recipe, using ingredients from all over the world to bring life and beauty to your skin. Couscous from North Africa rolls gently over the skin as cherimoya from South America softens and conditions. Southeast Asian water chestnuts not only exfoliate, but add their own natural moisture to your skin.

Use this terrific, tangy-smelling scrub weekly to gently lift old skin cells away and nourish and soften new skin, giving it a warm, radiant glow. If you happen to have extra-dry skin, try using it two or three times a week. If you have trouble finding the cherimoya or strawberry papaya in your market, try substituting a mango, which is loaded with vitamin A and softens skin beautifully.

For All Skin Types

Purpose: To gently exfoliate and cleanse the facial area.

Remember to do your patch test (page xiii).

couscous: exfoliant
cherimoya: conditioner
strawberry papaya: conditioner; A, C; papain
water chestnuts: exfoliant
baking soda: cleanser
buttermilk: conditioner; lactic acid
yogurt: conditioner; lactic acid
peas: conditioner; A, C
spinach: conditioner; A, C
anise: refresher; soother
watercress: healant

Botanical Formula

$1/2$ cup uncooked couscous

$1/4$ cherimoya (flesh and seeds)

$1/4$ strawberry papaya (flesh and seeds)

2 tablespoons chopped water chestnuts

2 tablespoons baking soda

2 tablespoons buttermilk

$1/2$ cup yogurt (use nonfat yogurt for oily skin)

9 pea pods (with peas)

2 chopped spinach leaves

$1/4$ cup chopped anise bulb or 1 teaspoon anise extract

2 tablespoons chopped watercress

Mix all ingredients together in a blender on medium speed for 2 to 4 minutes, or until smooth. Texture will be grainy because of the cherimoya seeds, water chestnuts, and couscous. Consistency should be smooth otherwise. Spread evenly onto face, scrubbing for 1 minute. Rinse with warm water and follow with a cleanser. If you save the remaining mixture, it will become softer as the couscous becomes hydrated. If you want more texture for future uses, blend another $1/2$ cup couscous in remaining mixture right before using. Makes 2 cups.

SHELF LIFE: Cover and refrigerate immediately; discard after 3 days.

Coco Palm
Facial Moisturizer

For Mature Skin

Purpose: To moisturize, condition, and soften mature skin.

Remember to do your patch test (page xiii).

vegetable oil: moisturizer

vegetable shortening: moisturizer

lemon juice: exfoliant; refresher; C

lime juice: exfoliant; refresher; C

coconut oil: moisturizer; scent

This moisturizer for mature skin is extremely simple to make and easy to use on a daily basis. Older skin constantly needs replenishment of moisture. The coconut oil or extract will leave a silky finish and sweet smell on your skin. If you prefer another flavor or scent, try strawberry or hazelnut extract, or your own personal favorite. A refreshing spritz of lemon and lime invigorates and excites the face. It also tightens and lifts skin, making wrinkles less apparent and the skin feel smoother and younger.

Botanical Formula

1 teaspoon vegetable oil

$^1/_3$ teaspoon vegetable shortening

1 teaspoon lemon juice

1 teaspoon lime juice

$^1/_3$ teaspoon coconut oil or extract

In a small saucepan, slowly heat ingredients together until warm. Remove from heat and let cool. Oils and juices will separate. Pour into a small cosmetic bottle and shake. Apply to face with a circular massaging motion. May be used on entire body. Makes 1 tablespoon.

SHELF LIFE: Store at room temperature; discard after 4 days.

Whipped Oatmeal–Sesame Seed Scrub Cream

If you have especially sensitive skin, you may be hesitating about using scrubs or exfoliators. Sensitive skin, however, needs to be conditioned on a regular basis, and that includes removal of dead skin cells. The key is to use a gentle product that will respect the sensitivity of your skin while also accomplishing the job for which it was designed.

   The consistency of this scrub is rich and thick. The soft abrasion will stimulate circulation and encourage new cell growth. Skin will be rosier and healthier, with a smooth satiny finish.

For Sensitive Skin

Purpose: To gently scrub and cleanse the face, remove dead skin cells, and condition skin.

Remember to do your patch test (page xiii).

baking soda: cleanser
whipping cream: moisturizer; softener
chamomile: healant; softener
cucumber: refresher
almond extract: emollient
lemon extract: emollient
pineapple extract: emollient
oatmeal: softener; exfoliant; B, E
sesame seeds: exfoliant; moisturizer

Botanical Formula

2 teaspoons baking soda

1/4 cup whipping cream

2 teaspoons chamomile

1/2 cucumber (do not peel)

1 teaspoon almond extract

1 teaspoon lemon extract

1 teaspoon pineapple extract

1 cup oatmeal

1/4 cup sesame seeds

FOR OILY SKIN:

Use skim milk instead of whipping cream

Omit almond and pineapple extracts

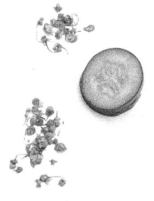

In a blender, mix all ingredients except for the oatmeal and sesame seeds on medium speed for 2 minutes. Place mixture in a bowl and stir in the oatmeal and sesame seeds, dispersing thoroughly. Apply to face with gentle circular motion, saturating skin with mixture. Rinse off with warm water. Follow with a toner and moisture. Use no more than 3 times a week. Makes 2 cups.

SHELF LIFE: Cover and refrigerate immediately; discard after 2 days.

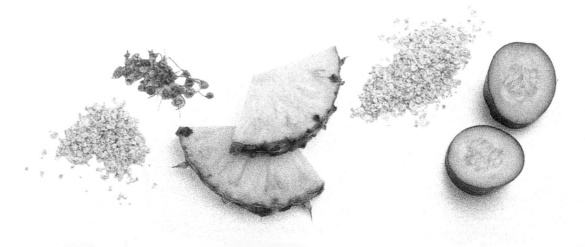

Strawberry-Almond Facial Scrub

For All Skin Types

Purpose: To gently exfoliate and cleanse the facial area, removing dead skin cells.

Remember to do your patch test (page xiii).

cucumber: cleanser; refresher

strawberries: cleanser; conditioner; C; iron; potassium

baking soda: cleanser

eggs: toner; ingredient binder

yogurt: conditioner; lactic acid

almonds: exfoliant

lemon juice: oil remover; **C**

Strawberries are truly one of nature's more sensual foods. The juicy, lush, red berry springs forth in May, bursting with tangy, sweet flavor. Whether fresh or frozen, this tantalizing fruit passes its own natural beauty on to you. While tickling the nose with their delicious aroma, the strawberries cleanse and condition the face, providing a light, astringent finish, as crushed almonds exfoliate and stimulate the skin.

The luscious, creamy texture of this scrub will coat and pamper your face, leaving it clean, revitalized, conditioned, and refreshed.

Botanical Formula

¹/₂ cup chopped cucumber
  (do not peel)

5 strawberries (hulled)

1 tablespoon baking soda

2 whole eggs

2 heaping tablespoons yogurt

²/₃ cup ground almonds

FOR DRY SKIN:

Use heavy cream instead of yogurt

FOR OILY SKIN:

Use nonfat yogurt instead

Add 2 teaspoons lemon juice

In a blender, puree the cucumber and strawberries together until smooth. Add baking soda, eggs, and yogurt and blend on medium-low speed for 20 seconds. Add the almonds and blend for 2 minutes on a pulse setting. Apply to moistened face in a gentle circular motion. Be sure to scrub gently, as too much pressure may be damaging to the skin. Rinse with warm water and again with cold water to close the pores. Pat face dry with a clean towel and follow with a cleanser. May be used daily. Makes 2 cups.

SHELF LIFE: Cover and refrigerate; discard after 3 days.

Honey-Oatmeal Facial Masque

Exfoliation on a regular basis is so important, but people with sensitive skin often have a hard time finding a product gentle enough. Oatmeal is a perfect match for this need. Richer in fat than other grains, oats replenish the skin with moisture, restoring softness and suppleness. It's no wonder they are used frequently in commercial soaps. Their gentle abrasion is great for any skin type, complemented by softeners of honey and yogurt, restoring suppleness and a healthy glow to your face.

NOTE: Apple seeds contain toxins—be sure to core your apple.

Botanical Formula

$^1/_2$ cup hot water

10 tablespoons quick oats

$^1/_2$ apple (cored, do not peel)

2 heaping tablespoons plain yogurt

2 tablespoons honey

1 egg white

Combine hot water and oats; stir until mixture is smooth. Let stand for 5 minutes, until water is absorbed completely and the mixture resembles a paste. Put the remaining ingredients into a blender and mix for 30 to 45 seconds. Then add oatmeal mixture and blend for another 10 to 20 seconds. For a thicker masque, add more oatmeal paste. Apply masque to entire face evenly and let sit for 10 to 15 minutes, until the skin begins to feel tight. Rinse thoroughly with warm water. Makes $^1/_2$ cup, enough for 1 application.

For Sensitive Skin

Purpose: To exfoliate sensitive skin and moisturize new skin layers.

Remember to do your patch test (page xiii).

oats: cleanser; exfoliant; D, E

apple: exfoliant; malic acid; A, C

yogurt: conditioner; lactic acid

honey: emollient

egg white: ingredient binder

Honey-Avocado Toning Masque

For Normal to Dry Skin

Purpose: To tone, cleanse, and tighten the skin.

Remember to do your patch test (page xiii).

avocado: moisturizer; A, C, D, E; potassium; thiamin; riboflavin
grapes: softener; A, C
egg: toner; ingredient binder
mayonnaise: conditioner
honey: emollient
baking soda: cleanser
lemon extract: refresher
lime extract: refresher

There is no disputing the fact that the avocado, with its 20% fat content, is a great moisturizer for skin. The lush, buttery flesh penetrates skin, giving it a healthy, moisture-rich glow. This masque utilizes the conditioning power of avocado along with grapes that soften and moisturize and mayonnaise, which tones and smoothes skin. Baking soda provides cleansing action gentle enough for even the most sensitive skin.

Botanical Formula

$^1/_2$ avocado (peeled and pitted)

3 seedless grapes

1 egg

1 teaspoon mayonnaise

1 teaspoon honey

1 tablespoon baking soda

1 teaspoon lemon extract

1 teaspoon lime extract

In a blender, puree the avocado, adding grapes one at a time. When smooth, add remaining ingredients and blend on medium speed for 45 seconds. This formula will not remain homogeneous; mix well before each application. Apply evenly to face, and leave on for 10 to 15 minutes, depending on desired toning. Makes $^1/_2$ cup.

SHELF LIFE: Cover and refrigerate immediately; discard after 3 days.

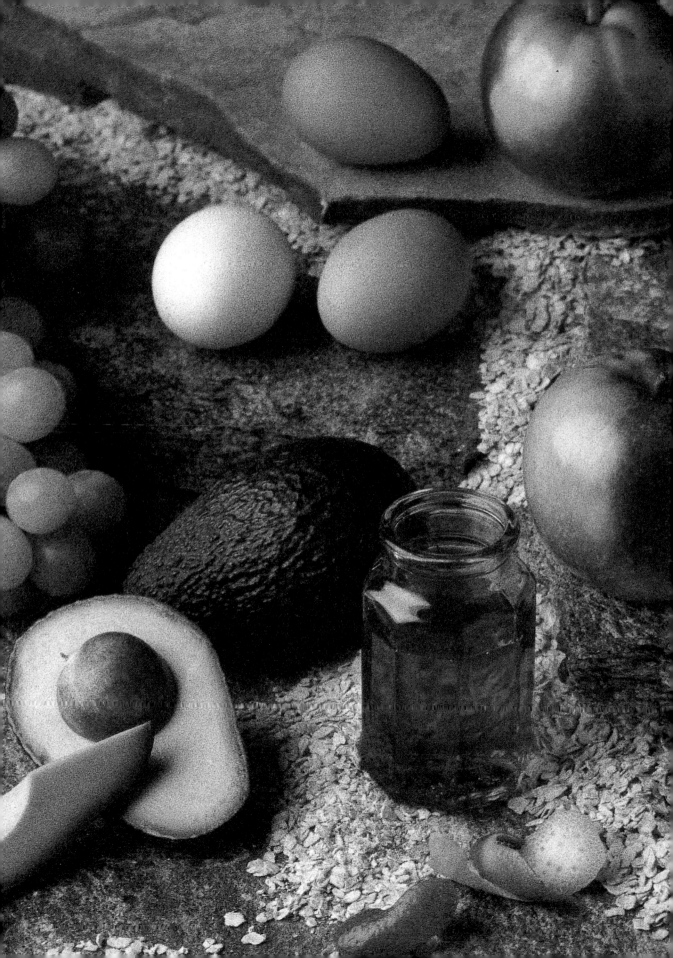

Napa Cabbage–Buttermilk Facial Slaw

For All Skin Types

*Purpose: To gently exfo-
liate and moisturize
skin.*

*Remember to do your
patch test (page xiii).*

**Napa cabbage: toner; A; folic
acid; potassium**

**buttermilk: moisturizer;
gentle exfoliator; lactic
acid**

**yogurt: moisturizer; exfo-
liant; lactic acid**

**eggs: toner; ingredient
binder**

**carrot: exfoliant; beta
carotene**

celery: astringent

**grapes: anti-inflammatory;
A, C; enzymes**

Napa cabbage, also known as Chinese cabbage, is a succulent, water-retaining leafy vegetable that works extremely well for cosmetic purposes. Its role in this facial slaw is primarily that of a gentle, cleansing refresher and toner. While it soothes the skin, it releases moisture, improving your face's tone and color.

Similar to cole slaw that you make at home, this facial slaw looks and smells delicious. Slather it on your face liberally, letting it settle in and thicken. You will feel the ingredients going to work, tightening, refreshing, and moisturizing. If you desire a thicker consistency, add another egg and double the yogurt.

Botanical Formula

1 cup chopped Napa cabbage

$^1/_4$ cup buttermilk

$^1/_4$ cup yogurt

2 whole eggs

1 chopped carrot (peeled)

2 stalks celery (no leaves)

10 white seedless grapes

FOR OILY SKIN:

Use nonfat yogurt

Use egg whites only; discard yolks

In a blender, mix all ingredients together on medium speed for 1 minute. Apply to face liberally, holding face up slightly until mixture sets. Let sit for 10 to 15 minutes. Rinse off with warm water. Use every other day, if possible. Makes 1$^1/_4$ cups.

SHELF LIFE: Cover and refrigerate; discard after 4 days.

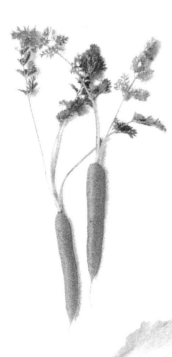

Facial Mist

Facial mists and atomizers are flooding the cosmetic counters. People are finally discovering that an all-day pickup for the face is available with a quick, cooling spritz. It wakes you up with an invigorating freshness. It penetrates and hydrates the skin and enhances your skin's color throughout the day.

This mist is perfect for any time of day. I recommend using a small hairspray bottle for a mister, because it's small enough to carry in a purse or briefcase. Simply wash out the bottle thoroughly, including the spray nozzle, fill it up, and you're ready to go. Spray it right on the face, even on top of makeup. It absorbs into the skin quickly, leaving a light, fresh scent behind.

For All Skin Types

Purpose: To moisten the face, prevent bacterial growth, and remove perspiration and dirt.

Remember to do your patch test (page xiii).

black tea: anti-inflammatory; refresher
hydrogen peroxide: antiseptic
lime extract: refresher; emollient

Botanical Formula

2 cups water

1 black tea bag

¹/₄ cup hydrogen peroxide (2.5% or less active)

1 teaspoon lime extract

Bring 1 cup of water to a boil, remove from heat, and immerse tea bag; let steep for 1 hour, as it cools. In a container, combine ¹/₄ cup of the brewed tea and 1 cup of water with hydrogen peroxide and lime extract. Pour into a spray bottle; shake gently to mix ingredients. Do not use if weather is cold or windy. Makes 1¹/₂ cups.

SHELF LIFE: Refrigerate; discard after 1 week.

Lemon-Lime Toner and Oil Remover

*For Moderately to Very
Oily Skin.*

*Purpose: To remove oil
from and tone the
skin.*

*Remember to do your
patch test (page xiii).*

**lemon juice: oil remover;
astringent; C**

**lime juice: oil remover;
astringent; C**

**apple cider vinegar: oil
remover**

**pineapple juice: anti-inflam-
matory; A, C; bromelain**

Although this toner can be used on any type skin, it is superb on extra-oily skin, which suffers year round, but especially in warmer weather. The astringency of lemon and lime lifts dirt from pores and gives a smoother appearance to the skin. This simple, refreshing formula is a great daily wake-up for the face. It should be used primarily in the t-zone of the face. This zone goes from the forehead down the nose and across the chin, and is the area of the face that is most susceptible to oil buildup. If fresh pineapple juice is not available, use juice from a can of chunk pineapple, but only the kind that is packed in natural juice, with no additional sugars.

Botanical Formula

1 tablespoon lemon juice

1 tablespoon lime juice

1 teaspoon apple cider vinegar

1 teaspoon pineapple juice

$^1/_4$ cup water

In a mixing bowl, combine all of the ingredients. Apply to the face with a cotton ball, blotting all over and concentrating on the t-zone. Toner should be applied after a cleanser and may be used every day for oily skin and every other day for moderately oily skin. It can also be used on the body if skin is oily. Makes 1/4 cup.

SHELF LIFE: Cover and refrigerate immediately; discard after 5 days.

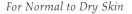

Cucumber-Parsley Facial Toner

Parsley has been used through the ages for medicinal purposes, from fever reducer to diuretic to skin healant, combatting disorders such as eczema and psoriasis. This familiar herb is available fresh year round, as are cucumbers, making this toner ideal for any time of the year. It can be used to refresh skin exhausted by warm weather as well as cold.

For Normal to Dry Skin

Purpose: To cleanse, tone, and refresh normal and dry complexion.

Remember to do your patch test (page xiii).

parsley: cleanser; A, C
potato: toner
cucumber: toner; astringent
almond extract: conditioner
lemon extract: astringent
lime extract: astringent

Botanical Formula

1 cup warm water

2 tablespoons chopped parsley

1/4 russet potato (scrubbed, do not peel)

1/4 cucumber (do not peel)

1 teaspoon almond extract

1 teaspoon lemon extract

1 teaspoon lime extract

In a small saucepan, bring water and parsley to a boil. Remove from heat and let cool slightly. Add to a blender and mix with other ingredients on medium speed for 30 seconds. Strain solution through a paper towel, saving liquid. Solids may be discarded. Saturate a cotton ball with the solution and apply to face, using a gentle dabbing motion. Use this after a scrub and cleanser. It is not necessary to rinse it off after use. Makes 1/2 cup.

SHELF LIFE: Cover and refrigerate; discard after 5 days.

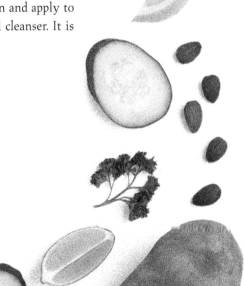

Bok Choy Facial Toner

For All Skin Types

Purpose: To tone and tighten skin.

Remember to do your patch test (page xiii).

mint leaves: stimulant; refresher

sage leaves: antiseptic; stimulant

fresh parsley: healant; A, C

thyme leaves: disinfectant

bok choy: refreshing toner

witch hazel: antiseptic; toner

lemon juice: oil remover; C

The crunchy, refreshing texture of bok choy is what inspired me to use it in a facial toner. A relative of Chinese cabbage, it's so gentle, and it possesses a natural astringency that refreshes and tones the skin. Using this toner daily will result in fresher, healthier-looking skin. When used following regular cleaning, it will lift residual dirt and oils, leaving pores cleaner and tighter. If you have oily skin, use this toner as the last step before applying makeup. Otherwise, follow it with a light moisturizer.

Botanical Formula

1 cup water

1 tablespoon chopped fresh mint leaves

2 sage leaves

$1/4$ cup chopped fresh parsley

2 tablespoons fresh thyme leaves

2 stalks bok choy (with leaves)

3 tablespoons witch hazel

FOR OILY SKIN:

Increase mint leaves to 2 tablespoons

Increase sage to 8 leaves

Increase witch hazel to 6 tablespoons

Add 1 tablespoon lemon juice

In a saucepan, heat water with mint, sage, parsley, and thyme; cover and simmer for 30 minutes. Remove from heat and let cool slightly. While still warm, pour infusion into a blender and mix with bok choy and witch hazel (and lemon juice for oily skin) and blend on medium speed for 2 minutes. Strain mixture through a coffee filter or paper towel, discarding the solids and saving the liquid. Using a cotton ball, apply liquid to face, blotting all over. Should be used after a cleanser. Makes $1^{1}/_{4}$ cups.

SHELF LIFE: Cover and refrigerate; discard after 4 days.

Witch Hazel–Vodka Conditioning Facial Toners

Starting with a solid base of vodka and witch hazel, these two toners take on the task of reviving skin and conditioning it after cleansing. Both formulas should be followed with a moisturizer, varying in intensity based on your skin type. After using the toner, however, your skin will already feel more refreshed and conditioned than with just a cleanser, and the tone and texture will be noticeably improved.

Botanical Formula

FOR DRY SKIN:

$^1/_4$ cup vodka

$^1/_4$ cup witch hazel

$^1/_4$ cup chopped cucumber (do not peel)

1 tablespoon olive oil

1 teaspoon canola oil

$^1/_8$ teaspoon orange oil or extract

FOR NORMAL SKIN:

$^1/_4$ cup vodka

1 teaspoon lemon juice

$^1/_4$ cup witch hazel

$^1/_4$ chopped cucumber (do not peel)

$^1/_4$ teaspoon alfalfa sprouts

$^1/_4$ teaspoon chopped mint leaves

1 teaspoon coconut extract

1 teaspoon almond extract

1 cup water

DIRECTIONS FOR DRY SKIN: In a blender, mix all ingredients together on low speed for 30 seconds. Store in a small cosmetic bottle. Apply to skin with a cotton ball. Mixture will not be homogeneous, so shake vigorously in bottle before every application. Makes $^1/_2$ cup.

DIRECTIONS FOR NORMAL SKIN: In a blender, mix all ingredients together on low speed for 45 seconds. Strain mixture through a coffee filter or paper towel, placing liquid in a small cosmetic bottle and discarding the solids. Apply with a cotton ball to the face. Makes $1^3/_4$ cups.

SHELF LIFE: Refrigerate immediately; discard after 5 days.

For Normal to Dry Skin

Purpose: To tone and tighten skin, reducing the size of pores while conditioning skin to prevent drying or chapping from cleansers.

Remember to do your patch test (page xiii).

vodka: astringent
witch hazel: astringent; healant
cucumber: refresher
olive oil: moisturizer
canola oil: moisturizer
orange oil or extract: moisturizer; scent
lemon juice: astringent; C
alfalfa sprouts: astringent; protein; minerals; C
mint leaves: invigorator
coconut extract: emollient
almond extract: emollient

Apricot and Wheat Germ Facial Moisturizing Masque

For Normal to Dry Skin

Purpose: To soften and smooth dry areas of skin.

Remember to do your patch test (page xiii).

avocados: moisturizer; A, C, D, E; potassium; thiamin; riboflavin

apricot: softener; conditioner; A

coconut milk: conditioner

wheat germ: conditioner; E

coconut oil: moisturizer; scent

honey: humectant

almond extract: emollient; scent

banana extract: emollient; scent

celery: astringent

egg white: toner

The apricot is one of summer's most delectable and delicate fruits. Highly perishable, this cousin of the peach hails originally from China, where it has been cultivated for centuries. The soft, sensual flesh of the apricot is fabulous for smoothing on skin for a rich conditioning treatment, enhanced with vitamin A. Combined with avocado, a rich, luscious softener in its own right, it creates a thick, creamy masque that hydrates skin, restoring moisture balance and softness.

Let the masque penetrate the skin thoroughly. After rinsing it away, you will notice a remarkable difference in your face. The color in your cheeks will be heightened, and the texture will be softer and silkier. Dry areas on the face will be healed and protected, feeling soothed and conditioned.

Botanical Formula

2 avocados (pitted and peeled)

¹/₂ apricot (pitted)

¹/₄ cup coconut milk

¹/₂ cup wheat germ

1 teaspoon coconut oil

1 teaspoon honey

1 teaspoon almond extract

1 teaspoon banana extract

1 stalk celery

1 egg white

In a blender, mix all ingredients on medium speed for 1 minute, or until smooth. After first cleansing skin, apply masque evenly on face and leave on for 15 minutes. Rinse off with warm water. Use 2 or 3 times a week for dry skin, once a week for normal skin. Makes 2 cups.

NOTE: After peeling the avocados, rub your knees and elbows with the inside of the peels. The abrasive texture exfoliates, and the flesh and oil of the avocado will provide softening to dry skin. Wipe off excess flesh and rub in oil until penetrated.

SHELF LIFE: Cover and refrigerate; discard after 3 days; avocado will turn dark green in container, but product will not be affected.

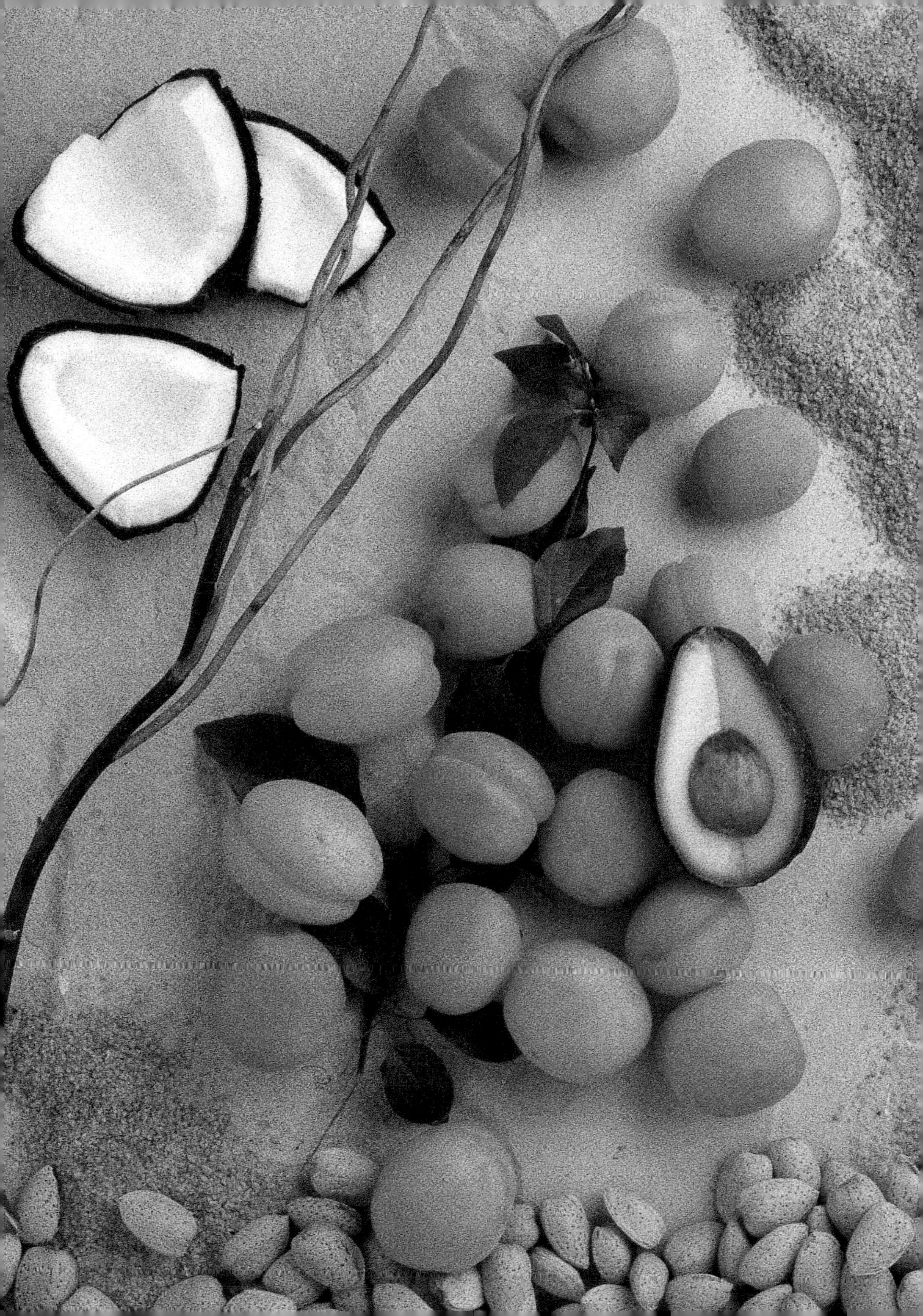

Ginger-Lemongrass After-Shave Lotion for Men

For All Skin Types

Purpose: To soothe and refresh the face after shaving.

Remember to do your patch test (page xiii).

ginger: antiseptic; stimulant
thyme: antiseptic; stimulant
lemongrass: cleanser; oil regulator
vegetable shortening: conditioner
lemon juice: astringent; C

Southeast Asia is full of bright colors and exotic sounds, heady aromas, and tastes. Two of the most dynamic food products commonly used in this region are lemongrass and ginger. Both ingredients play vital roles in this intriguing after-shave lotion.

Lemongrass is a cleansing facial herb that not only soothes skin irritations but also regulates overactive oil glands, creating more of an equilibrium on the skin's surface. It is also an antiseptic, creating a cleaner environment for the skin to flourish. Ginger, also an antiseptic, is a stimulating spice that invigorates skin and increases circulation. Daily use of this after-shave lotion will restore the skin to a healthier, cleaner state.

Botanical Formula

$^1/_2$ cup water

$^1/_{16}$ teaspoon (a small pinch) ground ginger*

3 whole stems thyme

2 tablespoons fresh lemongrass or 1 tablespoon dried

$^1/_2$ teaspoon vegetable shortening (use $^1/_4$ teaspoon for oily skin)

2 teaspoons lemon juice

Bring water to a boil and add ginger, thyme, and lemongrass. Simmer infusion for 30 minutes. Filter infusion with a coffee filter or paper towel, saving liquid and discarding solids. Return liquid to saucepan and add shortening and lemon juice. Mix over low heat, stirring until blended. Shortening will be separated from liquid. For future uses, mixture may be microwaved until slightly warm and stirred before using. Rub mixture into hands and spread over face, especially areas that have been shaved. May be used daily. Makes $^1/_4$ cup.

SHELF LIFE: Cover and refrigerate; discard after 5 days.

---

*Use caution when applying ginger to the skin. Start with a tiny pinch, and increase the amount just a bit if it does not irritate your skin.

Acorn Squash and Avocado Masque for Young Skin

Acorn squash is in plentiful supply throughout winter, and it's so great for the skin. A native of the Americas, this dark green, hard-shelled gourd is filled with vibrant yellow, starchy flesh that tones and rehydrates skin, in this case on younger bodies that experience increased wear and tear throughout the day.

Young skin should be taken care of as carefully as mature skin. A sense of youthful immortality leads many young men and women to ignore the realities of nature and the process of aging. This facial masque saturates skin with softeners that will help slow down wrinkle development in young skin. The creaminess of this masque makes it easy to apply. Your skin will feel renewed and toned, looking and feeling tighter and free of dry, dead skin cells. Follow with a moisturizer to lock in the conditioning powers that this masque delivers to your skin.

For All Skin Types

Purpose: To diminish appearance of wrinkles and try to prevent new wrinkling of the skin. This formula is not for mature skin.

Remember to do your patch test (page xiii).

avocado: moisturizer; A, C, D, E; potassium; thiamin; riboflavin
acorn squash: moisturizer; A
papaya: exfoliant; A, C; papain
lime: toner; C
lemon juice: toner; C
black tea: soother
alfalfa sprouts: astringent; protein; minerals; C
egg white: ingredient binder

Botanical Formula

2 avocados (pitted and peeled)

1 acorn squash (flesh only)

¹/₂ strawberry papaya or regular papaya

1 lime (peeled and seeded)

1 tablespoon lemon juice

2 tablespoons black tea

1 teaspoon alfalfa sprouts

1 egg white

In a blender, mix ingredients together on medium speed for 2 minutes, or until smooth. Cleanse skin first, then apply mixture evenly all over face. Leave on for 15 minutes. Wash off with warm water, and pat dry. Use up to 3 times a week for nonsensitive skin, less for sensitive skin. Makes 1³/₄ cups.

SHELF LIFE: Cover and refrigerate immediately, discard after 3 days.

Herbal Cleansing Milk for Men

For All Skin Types

Purpose: To cleanse and moisturize a man's face.

Remember to do your patch test (page xiii).

sage leaves: antiseptic; stimulant

rosemary leaves: antiseptic; stimulant

whole milk: cleanser; emollient; A, D

strawberries: cleanser; exfoliant; C; iron; potassium

baking soda: cleanser

cucumber: astringent

egg white: toner; ingredient binder

almond extract: emollient

lemon juice: oil remover; C

Men need to clean their skin as much as women do. After all, they collect the same dirt and bacteria in their skin. To create a balanced environment for masculine skin, try this cleansing milk every day. It conditions the skin, thoroughly cleanses it, and leaves it stimulated and smelling great.

Botanical Formula

$^1/_2$ cup water

1 tablespoon sage leaves

1 tablespoon rosemary leaves

$^1/_4$ cup whole milk

3 strawberries

2 tablespoons baking soda

$^1/_4$ cup chopped cucumber (do not peel)

1 egg white

1 tablespoon almond extract

FOR OILY SKIN:

Use skim milk instead of whole milk

Omit almond extract

Add 1 tablespoon lemon juice

Bring water, sage, and rosemary leaves to a boil. Simmer for 30 minutes, making an infusion. In a blender, mix infusion (water and herbs) with remaining ingredients on medium speed for 30 seconds, or until smooth. Wet face with warm water; apply mixture to face with a washcloth, scrubbing gently in a circular motion. Rinse with warm water. Follow with toner. Makes 1 cup.

SHELF LIFE: Cover and refrigerate immediately; discard after 4 days.

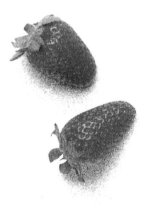

Refreshing Beer Masque for Men

Men's skin is often overlooked in beauty circles, but skin needs to be conditioned and looked after, no matter what sex you are. Beer is a great softener for skin, and it smells great in this masque.

Botanical Formula

1 tablespoon beer

1 heaping teaspoon yogurt

1 teaspoon olive oil

1 egg white

1 teaspoon lemon extract

1 teaspoon almond extract

FOR OILY SKIN:

Add 1/2 teaspoon lemon juice

Use nonfat yogurt

In a blender, mix all ingredients together on low speed for 20 to 30 seconds. When mixture is smooth, wet the facial area with warm water, then apply mixture to skin evenly. Leave on the skin for 15 to 20 minutes. Rinse with warm water. When completely rinsed off, splash face with cold water to seal pores. Makes 1/4 cup.

SHELF LIFE: Cover and refrigerate immediately; discard after 2 days.

For All Skin Types

Purpose: To soothe, moisturize, and soften the facial area.

Remember to do your patch test (page xiii).

beer: softener
yogurt: softener; lactic acid
olive oil: conditioner
egg white: toner
lemon extract: refresher
almond extract: emollient
lemon juice: astringent; C

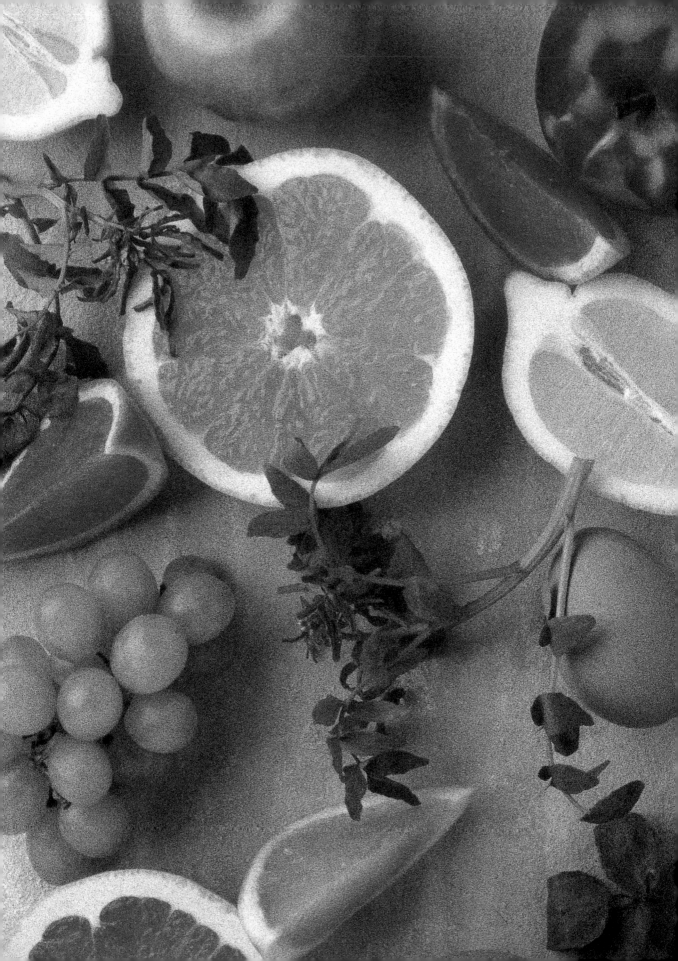

Apple-Grapefruit Acne Masque

The grapefruit is a relative newcomer to the food world compared to ancient grains and herbs. It was developed toward the late 18th century as a hybrid of pomelo, another tropical citrus fruit, and an orange, and is great for skin with acne, which experiences overactive oil production, blocking pores with excess skin cells, as well as dirt and bacteria. The grapefruit's citric acid helps to remove oil on the surface of the skin and penetrate pores

If you have a high grade of acne, you may be on an antibiotic. It is still important, however, to maintain a clean, healthy environment in which your skin can thrive. Regular exfoliation and oil removal help new skin breathe and flourish, giving your face a chance to look and feel great.

NOTE: Apple seeds contain toxins—be sure to core your apple.

Botanical Formula

¹/₄ grapefruit (seeded and peeled)

¹/₄ lemon (seeded and peeled)

¹/₄ apple (cored, do not peel)

20 green seedless grapes

3 tablespoons chopped watercress

1 egg white

Blend all ingredients together on medium speed for 2 minutes, or until pureed. Apply gently to the face and leave on for 15 to 30 minutes. Rinse with warm water and softly blot dry. Makes 1 cup.

SHELF LIFE: Store and refrigerate immediately; discard after 3 to 5 days.

For Skin with Acne

Purpose: To cleanse acne-affected skin, removing dead cells encased around the acne and leaving the skin feeling softer.

Remember to do your patch test (page xiii).

grapefruit: exfoliant; astringent; citric acid; C

lemon: exfoliant; astringent; C

apple: exfoliant; malic acid; A, C

grapes: anti-inflammatory; A, C

watercress: healant

egg white: toner

White Wine and Mint Blemish Treatment Masque

For All Skin Types

Purpose: To deeply cleanse blemished areas.

Remember to do your patch test (page xiii).

white wine: oil remover
lemon juice: astringent; oil remover; C
lime juice: astringent; oil remover; C
mint leaves: stimulant
cucumber: refresher
watercress: healant; oil remover

The alcohol in white wine makes it a fast-drying, effective ingredient that, along with other oil reducers and healants, creates a more balanced environment for the face. Blemishes are discouraged from forming, and existing blemishes are medicated and begin the healing process. Your face will look and feel refreshed, invigorated, and cleansed of heavy, dirty oil buildup.

Botanical Formula

2 tablespoons dry white wine*

1 teaspoon lemon juice

1 teaspoon lime juice

1 teaspoon mint leaves

$1/2$ cucumber (do not peel)

3 tablespoons chopped watercress

In a blender, mix all ingredients together on medium speed for 45 seconds, or until smooth. Apply to the face, patting lightly with fingers; leave on for 15 minutes. Rinse with warm water and follow with a cleanser. May be used every other day. Makes $3/4$ cup.

SHELF LIFE: Cover and refrigerate; discard after 5 days.

---

*Use a chardonnay or dry white wine; avoid sweeter wines with residual sugars.

Apple and Watercress Blemish Treatment Masque

The soft mash of apple and potato gives this blemish masque a wonderfully thick texture that embraces and caresses the face. As the masque penetrates the skin, it draws oil and dirt out of the pores, lifting them to the surface to be washed away. Irritations and blemishes begin healing with the help of watercress, which soothes and medicates pores. The potato also helps reduce swelling of tissue, especially areas inflamed by blemishes. Refreshed and invigorated, your face will look and feel cleaner. Texture and resiliency of skin is improved and a fresher, less irritated appearance will emerge. Pores will be less noticeable as the skin is toned and tightened with a smoother, matte finish.

NOTE: Apple seeds contain toxins—be sure to core your apple.

Botanical Formula

$^1/_2$ chopped apple (cored, do not peel)

3 tablespoons watercress

1 tablespoon lemon juice

1 tablespoon lime juice

$^1/_4$ chopped potato (do not peel)

$^1/_2$ cucumber (do not peel)

1 tablespoon mint leaves

2 egg whites

In a blender, mix all ingredients together on medium speed for 45 seconds, or until mixture is smooth. Apply to face evenly with fingers. Leave on for 15 to 20 minutes. Rinse with warm water, then rinse again with cool water. Use 3 times a week. Makes 1 cup.

SHELF LIFE: Cover and refrigerate immediately; discard after 5 days.

For Oily Skin

Purpose: To remove dirt and oil from blemished skin; to improve softness in skin.

Remember to do your patch test (page xiii).

apple: exfoliant; malic acid; A, C
watercress: healant; oil remover
lemon juice: astringent; oil remover; C
lime juice: astringent; oil remover; C
potato: toner
cucumber: refresher
mint leaves: stimulant
egg whites: toner; ingredient binder

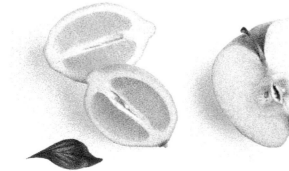

Celery and Alfalfa Sprout Blemish Cream Treatment

For All Skin Types

Purpose: To dry blemishes and pimples and to remove blackheads.

Remember to do your patch test (page xiii).

mint leaves: stimulant
watercress: healant
celery: toner; healant
alfalfa sprouts: astringent; protein; minerals; **C**
apple: exfoliant; malic acid; **A, C**

The astringency of pureed celery is perfect for a blemish treatment. As the apple in this formula lifts off dead skin cells, the celery and alfalfa sprouts tighten and tone skin, reducing the appearance of pores and resulting in an overall smooth texture. Celery also medicates and heals pores.

The light consistency and gentleness of this cream make it ideal for any type of skin. Follow it with a toner and light moisturizer.

NOTE: Apple seeds contain toxins—be sure to core the apple.

Botanical Formula

1 cup water

1 teaspoon mint leaves

3 tablespoons watercress

1 celery stalk, chopped (no leaves)

1 teaspoon alfalfa sprouts

1 apple (cored and chopped, do not peel)

Bring water, mint, and watercress to a boil; reduce heat and simmer infusion for 30 minutes. In a blender, mix $1/2$ cup of infusion with other ingredients on medium speed for 1 minute, or until smooth. Apply to face, patting on gently; leave on for 15 minutes. Rinse well with warm water. May be used daily. Makes 1 cup.

SHELF LIFE: Cover and refrigerate; discard after 3 days.

Sesame-Cucumber Facial Line Reducer

The face is such a sensitive area, reacting strongly to chemicals, weather, diet, and, of course, the amount of sleep you get each time. A night out filled with smoke, alcohol, and not enough rest can result in increased lines around the eyes, giving your face an older, wearier appearance. Sesame oil is a fabulous soothing ointment for the face. It has been used cosmetically for centuries on all types of skin. It is gentle even on sensitive skin, which is imperative, especially when dealing with the eye area, and it leaves a soft, silky finish as it is absorbed into the skin.

This formula will not erase permanent lines around your eyes due to aging or other factors, such as overexposure to sun. It will, however, temporarily diminish the appearance of these lines and will help erase lines associated with lack of sleep and exposure to harmful elements. Not only will your eye area look smoother and more refreshed, it will feel less puffy and stressed.

For All Skin Types

Purpose: To cosmetically reduce the appearance of lines around the eyes.

Remember to do your patch test (page xiii).

cucumber: refresher; astringent
potato: toner
chamomile tea: healant
egg whites: toner; ingredient binder
light sesame oil: emollient

Botanical Formula

¹/₂ cup chopped cucumber (do not peel)

¹/₂ cup russet potato (scrubbed, do not peel)

3 tablespoons chamomile tea

2 egg whites

2 tablespoons light sesame oil

In a blender, mix all of the ingredients on medium speed for 45 seconds, or until smooth. Apply on area around eyes, concentrating on lines. Leave on for 15 to 20 seconds, then rinse with lukewarm water. For additional applications, whisk formula by hand in a small bowl and apply as usual. Use 2 to 3 times a week. Makes 1¹/₂ cups.

SHELF LIFE: Cover and refrigerate immediately; discard after 3 or 4 days.

Herbal Carrot Blemish Treatment

For All Skin Types

Purpose: To treat blemishes on the face caused by pimples.

Remember to do your patch test (page xiii).

parsley: healant; A, C
mint leaves: stimulant
watercress: healant; oil remover
carrots: healant; beta carotene
egg white: toner; ingredient binder

Carrots are great for sores, especially blemishes on the face. They gently medicate and cleanse the pores and surface of the skin, providing soothing, antiseptic relief.

Whipped into this light, creamy mixture, carrots work with their companions to begin the process of healing infected, blemished skin. Pores will be left free of excess oil and cleaner, inside and out. Using this treatment every other day will help rid your skin of existing blemishes and discourage future irritations from occurring.

Botanical Formula

1 cup water

¹/₄ cup parsley

1 tablespoon mint leaves

¹/₄ cup watercress

3 medium-size carrots (peeled and chopped)

1 egg white

Bring water, parsley, mint, and watercress to a boil; reduce heat and simmer for 30 minutes. Remove from heat and let cool. In a blender, mix infusion with carrots and egg white on medium speed for 45 seconds. Apply to face by patting on gently; let sit for 10 to 20 minutes. Rinse off with warm water. Cleanse face first; after treatment, follow with toner and moisturizer. Makes 1¹/₄ cups.

SHELF LIFE: Cover and refrigerate immediately; discard after 3 days.

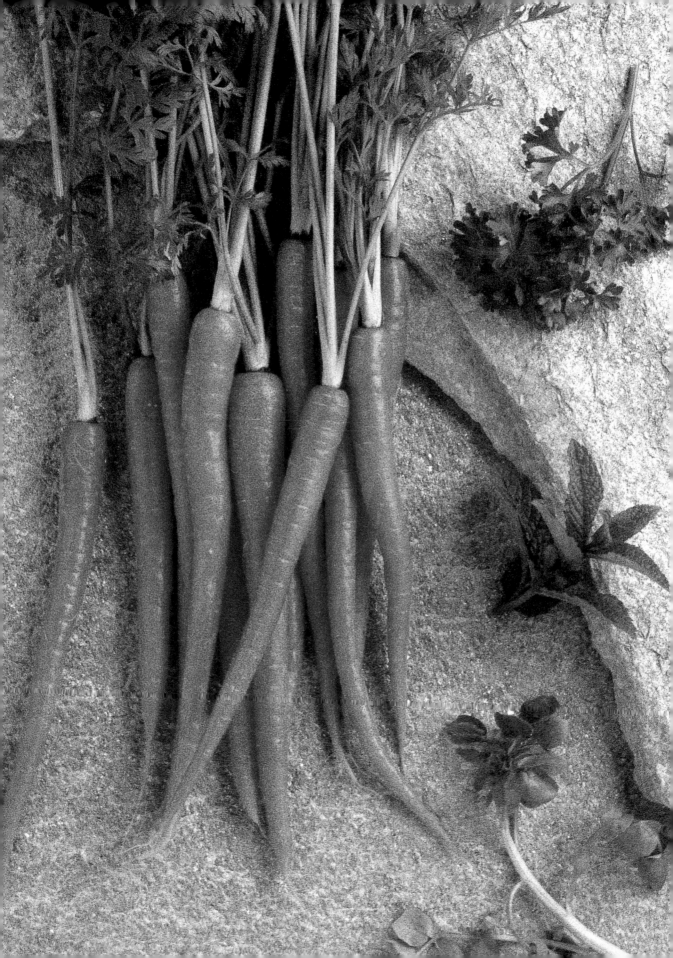

Soft and Gentle
Eye Makeup Remover

For All Skin Types

*Purpose: To remove
makeup around the
eyes.*

*Remember to do your
patch test (page xiii).*

canola oil: solvent
castor oil: solvent
olive oil: solvent
avocado oil: emollient

Castor oil is a highly valued ingredient in cosmetics. It is terrific for removing makeup, especially the more stubborn products, such as mascara.

Botanical Formula

1 tablespoon canola oil

1 tablespoon castor oil

1 tablespoon olive oil

1 teaspoon avocado oil

In a small cosmetic bottle, combine all of the ingredients. Shake gently to mix thoroughly. Apply to eye area with a cotton ball. Avoid getting formula into eyes. The makeup will be wiped clean instantly.

SHELF LIFE: Store at room temperature; discard after 5 days.

Chamomile-Fig
Eye and Facial Soother

Our eyes take a daily beating, with exposure to harmful elements making them puffy and swollen. This formula uses the soothing and anti-inflammatory properties of figs, chamomile, and black tea to reduce this swelling, restoring skin around the eyes to its proper proportions and leaving your eyes feeling refreshed and pampered.

I recommend using this soother several times a day. By the end of the day, you will notice a significant change in the way skin around your eyes looks.

For All Skin Types

Purpose: To reduce puffiness and swelling around the eyes.

Remember to do your patch test (page xiii).

black tea: soother
chamomile tea: anti-inflammatory
fig: anti-inflammatory; iron; calcium; phosphorous
cucumber: refresher; astringent
potato: toner

Botanical Formula

$^1/_2$ cup water

1 black tea bag

3 chamomile tea bags or 3 tablespoons loose tea

$^1/_2$ fig

$^1/_4$ cucumber (do not peel)

1 russet potato (scrubbed and chopped, do not peel)

Bring water to a boil; remove from heat and add all 4 tea bags or black tea bag and loose chamomile. Steep for $^1/_2$ hour. Remove tea bags and strain if necessary to remove loose chamomile. In a blender, mix $^1/_4$ cup of the tea with fig, cucumber, and potato on medium speed for 45 seconds. Apply gently with one finger around the eyes and leave for 5 to 10 minutes. Rinse off with warm water. Makes 1$^1/_4$ cups.

SHELF LIFE: Cover and refrigerate; discard after 4 days.

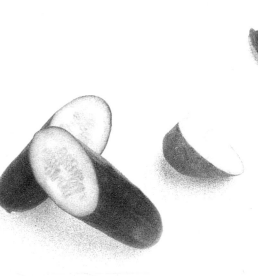

Watercress and Rice
Acne Facial Toner

For Oily Skin and Skin with Acne

Purpose: To tone, refresh, and treat skin with excess oil or acne.

Remember to do your patch test (page xiii).

watercress: healant
rice: toner; tightener
lemon juice: astringent; oil remover; C
grapes: anti-inflammatory; A, C

Acne takes a tremendous toll on skin. The presence of excess oil, skin cells, and bacteria building up in the pores, causing redness and swelling, leaves the skin looking rough and less toned that it should be, not to mention potential scarring. A facial toner will not stop acne from occurring. It will, however, improve the look and feel of your skin with regular use. As the skin cells die, they build up on the surface of the skin, so it's important to cleanse thoroughly, removing the excess cells and oil, and to follow with an astringent toner.

Botanical Formula

2 cups water

3 tablespoons chopped watercress

$1/_2$ cup long-grain rice

$1/_4$ cup lemon juice

10 green seedless grapes

Bring water and watercress to a light boil; remove from heat, add rice to mixture, stir together, and let steep for 30 minutes. In a blender, mix watercress, water, and rice with lemon juice and grapes on medium-low speed for 45 seconds, or until pureed. Then strain mixture through a paper towel or coffee filter. If particles still remain in the liquid, filter again. Product should be filtrate free. Apply to face all over with a cotton ball. Do not rinse off. Use every day. Makes 2 cups.

SHELF LIFE: Cover and refrigerate immediately; discard after 4 days.

Watercress-Papaya Acne Cleanser

Watercress is carefully cultivated these days, but it can also be found growing wild in gentle streams in the countryside. This spicy, flavorful member of the mustard family has natural healing properties that work beautifully with acne-plagued skin, cleaning oil and dirt from inside and around the pores. This cleanser will not cure your acne, but it will help you maintain a better tone and texture. Your newly revealed skin will glow with a healthy color, your complexion will be improved, and your face will feel smoother and softer to the touch.

NOTE: Apple seeds contain toxins—be sure to core your apple.

Botanical Formula

5 tablespoons chopped watercress

1/2 strawberry papaya

1/2 cored apple (do not peel)

1/2 lemon (seeded and peeled)

1/2 teaspoon chopped basil leaves

6 green seedless grapes

1/4 teaspoon orange extract

1/4 teaspoon lemon extract

5 tablespoons baking soda*

1 cup water

In a blender, mix all ingredients except the baking soda and water on medium speed for 30 seconds, or until pureed. In a separate container, combine the baking soda and water, mixing by hand until baking soda is dissolved. Add baking soda solution to blender and mix with existing solution on low for 10 seconds. Gently apply to face with a firm, circular motion, penetrating skin thoroughly; rinse with warm water. Pat face dry softly. Makes 1³/4 cups.

SHELF LIFE: Cover and refrigerate immediately; discard after 3 days.

---

*If skin dries out too much after using, reduce baking soda to 2 tablespoons.

For Skin with Acne

Purpose: To cleanse skin with acne, deeply penetrating to remove dead skin cells and improve the surface of the skin.

Remember to do your patch test (page xiii).

watercress: healant
strawberry papaya: exfoliant; A, C; papain
apple: exfoliant; malic acid; A, C
lemon: astringent; C
basil leaves: pain reliever; stimulant
grapes: anti-inflammatory; A, C
orange extract: emollient
lemon extract: emollient
baking soda: cleanser

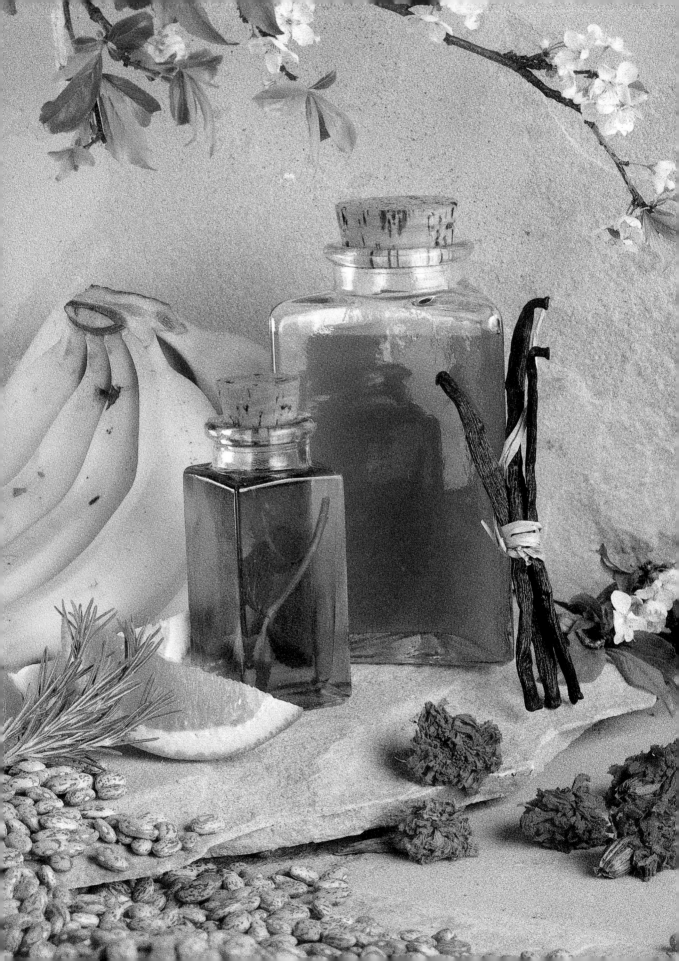

Hair Care

Hair Care

HAIR IS SUCH A BIG PART OF BEAUTY. Your hairstyle can make you or break you. The key is to work with your stylist to discover what style is right for you. It takes time to develop the right look, and it involves choices, some of which may go against the tide of fashion but may be right for you.

Not only is the cut important, but also the quality and color of the hair. I often encounter women who want to change their hairstyle and color after a relationship has ended. I don't recommend changing color, however, unless you are committed to maintaining it. Healthy hair grows an average of half an inch per month, and touchup of roots can become tiresome. What I do recommend is working to enhance your natural hair color with rinses and highlighters. For example, I developed the Black Tea–Rosemary Rinse to restore a rich, dark tone to dark hair, bringing out the hair's natural luster while neutralizing excess red tones.

This chapter contains recipes for all aspects of hair care and for all types of hair. Use a mixture of vodka, apple juice, and orange extract to remove buildup of hair care products before shampooing. Spray your hair with citrus juice before sunning for a natural hair lightener. Make a deep conditioning treatment by whirling coconut milk, sesame oil, and honey in your blender. Or add coconut milk, macadamia nut oil, and mayonnaise to your favorite shampoo for a tropical shampoo and conditioner in one.

By using natural hair care products that you have made yourself, you can boost the beauty and luster of your hair with formulas that contain a much higher degree of active ingredients than commercial formulas.

> *Stand on the highest pavement of the stair—*
>
> *Lean on a garden urn—*
>
> *Weave, weave the sunlight in your hair.*
>
> —T.S. ELIOT

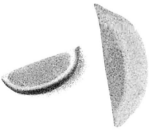

Lemony Rum Buildup Remover
with Shampoo

For All Hair Types

Purpose: To enhance your regular shampoo with elements that remove hair product buildup without stripping hair of proteins.

Remember to do your patch test (page xiii).

shampoo: cleanser
apple juice: buildup remover; scalp exfoliant
lemon extract: buildup remover
rum extract: oil remover
lemon juice: shine; C

If you have ever been to the Caribbean and sat on the beach watching a glorious sunset, you should definitely try this recipe. Close your eyes and let the fragrance of rum carry you back to a tropical setting with calm waters and easier days. Once called "sugar wine," rum is distilled from sugar cane or molasses, and has no doubt tickled your tastebuds, from piña coladas to daiquiris, from the tropics to your home.

This formula uses rum extract as an oil remover for hair that has experienced a heavy buildup of hair products, such as mousses, conditioners, sprays, and gels, which attract oil as well. Apple juice and lemon extract also act as buildup removers. All of these elements are incorporated into a one-step cleansing formula that lets you pick your own cleanser.

I recommend using this formula at least once a week, depending on the number of hair products you use. If you use one to several products a day, beyond those for shampooing and conditioning, you may need to use it more often.

Botanical Formula

$^1/_4$ cup shampoo*

$1^1/_2$ tablespoons apple juice

$^1/_2$ teaspoon lemon extract

$^1/_2$ teaspoon rum extract

$1^1/_2$ tablespoons lemon juice

In a mixing bowl, whisk together all ingredients until blended. Formula will foam up slightly. Shampoo hair with mixture, let sit for 5 minutes, and rinse.

SHELF LIFE: Cover and refrigerate; discard after 3 days.

*Commercial shampoo should not be a one-step shampoo (with conditioner), a dandruff shampoo, or an oily hair shampoo.

Rum and Egg Buildup Remover
with Shampoo

The combination of rum and eggs is one of the oldest hair care recipes around. Here they are used as a shampoo additive to remove oil and hair product buildup on your hair. Paired with the egg and rum is peppermint extract, a great-smelling addition that also removes oil. Once the oil and buildup have been removed, the shampoo of your choice cleanses them away. After shampooing, your hair will feel and look cleaner, with a soft, healthy shine and fabulous minty scent.

For Normal to Oily Hair

Purpose: To remove oil buildup on hair and restore body.

Remember to do your patch test (page xiii).

shampoo: cleanser
white rum: oil remover
egg: softener
peppermint extract: oil remover; scent

Botanical Formula

1 cup shampoo*

1 tablespoon white rum

1 whole egg

1 teaspoon peppermint extract

In a blender, mix all ingredients together on low speed for 30 to 40 seconds, or until completely mixed. Mixture will foam slightly. Shampoo as usual, and rinse with warm water. Makes 1 cup.

SHELF LIFE: Cover and refrigerate; discard after 5 days.

---

*Commercial shampoo should not be a one-step shampoo (with conditioner), a dandruff shampoo, or an oily hair shampoo.

Vanilla-Rum Cocktail

For Oily Hair

Purpose: To soften hair and remove oil deposits on hair; to add shine and manageability.

Remember to do your patch test (page xiii).

white rum: oil remover
beer: softener; volumizer
eggs: softener
lemon extract: oil remover
vanilla extract: softener

Rum is a marvelous remedy for oily deposits found on hair and scalp. Pure silver or deep, amber gold, it cuts right through the buildup, lifting the oils and dirt away, leaving cleaner, healthier hair. The sweet, warm fragrance of vanilla accents this weekly treatment for oily hair, leaving it baby fine and soft to the touch.

Botanical Formula

$^1/_2$ *cup white rum*

$^1/_2$ *cup beer (not light beer)*

2 whole eggs

$^1/_2$ *teaspoon lemon extract*

$^1/_2$ *teaspoon vanilla extract*

$^1/_2$ *cup warm water*

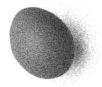

In a blender, mix all ingredients on medium speed for 20 seconds. Massage mixture through hair right down to the scalp. Mixture will foam up a bit with massaging. Leave on for up to 5 minutes. Rinse with warm water. Follow with regular shampooing. Makes 1$^3/_4$ cups.

SHELF LIFE: Cover and refrigerate; discard after 2 days.

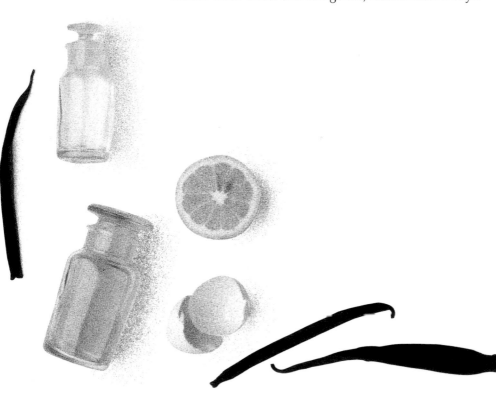

Preshampooing Orange-Vodka Buildup Remover

Vodka's very nature—astringent and dry—makes it ideal for reducing buildup on hair. This buildup remover, meant to be sprayed on before shampooing, penetrates and clarifies the hair shaft, allowing its natural highlights to shine through.

Botanical Formula

$1/_4$ cup vodka

2 tablespoons apple juice

2 tablespoons apple cider vinegar

1 teaspoon lemon extract

1 teaspoon orange extract

In a blender, mix all ingredients on medium speed for 20 seconds. The mixture will not be completely homogeneous. Just mix enough to disperse the oils. Pour mixture into a spray bottle, shake, and spray onto the hair. Use this product before shampooing and conditioning. Makes $1/4$ cup.

SHELF LIFE: Refrigerate immediately; discard after 5 days.

For Normal to Oily Hair

Purpose: To remove buildup of hair products without completely drying out the hair or stripping hair of natural oils.

Remember to do your patch test (page xiii).

vodka: stripping agent; astringent
apple juice: stripping agent
apple cider vinegar: clarifier
lemon extract: scent
orange extract: scent

Honey-Maple Hot Oil Treatment

For Normal to Dry Hair

Purpose: To deeply condition, strengthen, and soften hair, adding body and shine.

Remember to do your patch test (page xiii).

canola oil: conditioner
margarine: conditioner
olive oil: conditioner
coconut oil: scent
orange oil: scent
light sesame oil: conditioner
macadamia nut oil: conditioner
avocado oil: conditioner
maple syrup: humectant
honey: humectant

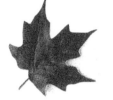

Whether it's the middle of a brutally cold winter or a scorching summer, hair has a tendency to dry out on us. A regular hair care regime including hot oil treatments is vital for the life and luster of your hair. Once you have split ends, you might as well cut them off. However, a deep, penetrating combination of oils and softeners can revitalize hair and restore it to a luxurious, shiny, healthy state. Use this treatment whenever your feel your hair is drying out, especially if you are prone to dry skin or hair. Only use this treatment warm because the oils become thinner when heated and penetrate the hair shaft and scalp more easily.

Botanical Formula

1 teaspoon canola oil

1 teaspoon margarine (softened)

1 tablespoon olive oil

1 teaspoon coconut oil*

1 teaspoon orange oil*

1 tablespoon light sesame oil

1 teaspoon macadamia nut oil

1 teaspoon avocado oil

¹/₂ teaspoon maple syrup

¹/₄ teaspoon honey

In a saucepan on low heat, mix all of the ingredients together except for the syrup and honey. When they are warm and mixed well, remove from heat. Cool slightly and add syrup and honey. Make sure it is not too hot to apply to scalp. Massage warm mixture through hair thoroughly and leave on for 10 to 20 minutes, depending on dryness. For best results, cover hair with plastic. Rinse with warm water and follow with a shampoo. Makes ¹/₄ cup, enough for one application.

---

*If coconut oil and orange oil are not available, use extracts.

Preventative Dandruff Treatment

This formula is great for extra help in combatting the effects of dandruff. Apple juice by itself soaks into the hair and scalp, giving intensive exfoliation and relief to dry flakiness. Use the juice and rinse every other day for a week after shampooing and conditioning. It remains on the hair and should provide significant relief after two or three uses. After the first week, use it once a week, or more often as needed.

For All Hair Types

Purpose: To reduce dandruff.

Remember to do your patch test (page xiii).

apple juice: exfoliant
apple cider vinegar: dandruff reducer

Botanical Formula

TREATMENT:

1 cup fresh apple juice

RINSE:

2 teaspoons apple cider vinegar

1 cup water

Massage apple juice treatment throughout the hair, saturating hair shafts, scalp, and follicles. Combine rinse ingredients in a cup, stirring together. Rinse hair with this solution.

Vegetarian Refried Bean Hair Masque

For Normal to Dry Hair

Purpose: To soften and add shine and volume to hair.

Remember to do your patch test (page xiii).

refried beans: moisturizer; protein
avocado: moisturizer; A, C, D, E; potassium; thiamin; riboflavin
Brussels sprouts: moisturizer; A, C, D; iron
coconut milk: fortifier
sweet potatoes: fortifier; A, C
macadamia nut oil: softener
olive oil: softener
canola oil: softener

The smooth consistency of refried beans provides a marvelous base for a hair masque. It is thick and easy to manage and bonds well with hair. Plus, it provides essential moisture to dried or damaged hair because of its high fat content. This masque smells great, feels fabulous while it's on, and is so much fun to put together. Its creamy thickness coats and soothes the head, feeding the hair and scalp and restoring moisture and strength.

Botanical Formula

¹/₂ cup refried beans (vegetarian— no animal fats)

¹/₂ avocado (peeled, pitted)

8 cooked Brussels sprouts (fresh or frozen)

¹/₄ cup coconut milk

2 tablespoons chopped cooked sweet potatoes (fresh or frozen)

2 tablespoons macadamia nut oil

2 tablespoons olive oil

2 tablespoons canola oil

In a blender, mix all ingredients together on medium-low speed for 45 seconds. When the formula is smooth, apply by massaging through the hair, and cover with a plastic cap or plastic wrap. Leave on hair for 10 to 20 minutes, then rinse thoroughly with warm water until mixture is completely gone. Removal of masque may take scrubbing action during rinse. Makes 2 cups.

SHELF LIFE: Cover and refrigerate; discard after 2 days.

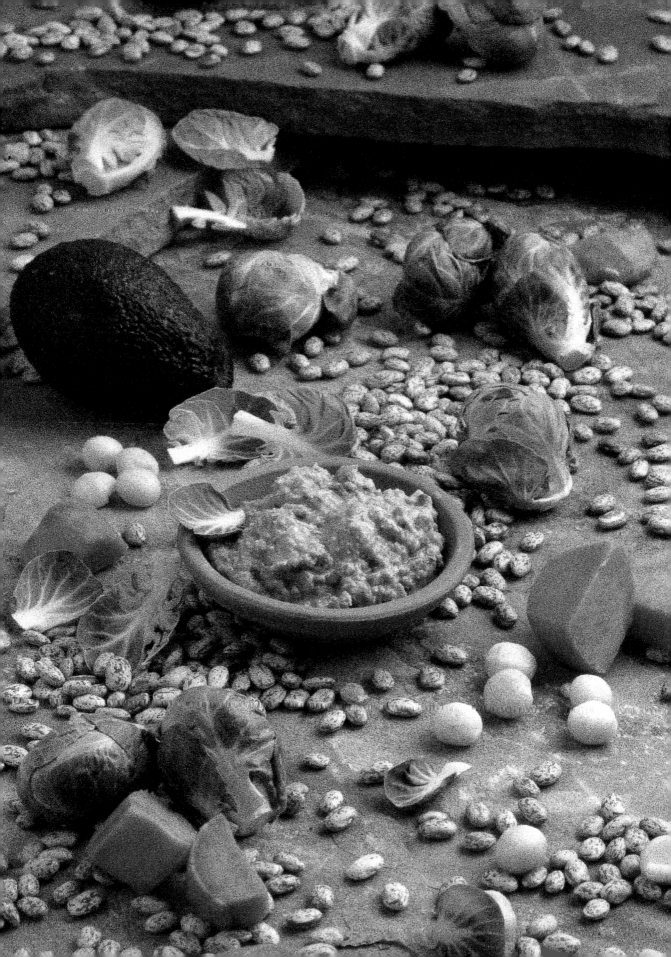

Sesame-Coconut Protein Conditioner

For Normal to Dry Hair

*Purpose: To reduce brit-
tleness and increase
softness and manage-
ability of hair.*

*Remember to do your
patch test (page xiii).*

olive oil: conditioner
light sesame oil: conditioner
eggs: softener
coconut milk: volumizer
honey: softener
coconut oil: scent

Both sesame and olive oil provide a moisture seal in this thick, luxurious hair conditioner. They nourish and rehydrate the scalp and hair strands and restore luster and shine to dry, brittle hair.

Botanical Formula

2 tablespoons olive oil

2 tablespoons light sesame oil

2 whole eggs

2 tablespoons coconut milk

2 tablespoons honey

1 teaspoon coconut oil

In a blender, mix all ingredients together on low speed for 30 seconds, or until smooth. Mixture will foam up a bit because of the eggs. Shampoo as usual and rinse. Then apply mixture to hair, massaging it in with fingers or a comb. Leave on for up to 5 minutes, then rinse with warm water. May be used daily and left on longer for more intensive conditioning. Makes ³/₄ cup.

SHELF LIFE: Cover and refrigerate immediately; discard after 5 days.

Polynesian One-Step Shampoo and Conditioner

This formula reflects the growing need for one-step shampoo conditioners. The one-step products have flooded the market and are designed as time savers, putting the steps of shampooing and conditioning into one. While I advocate their use, I don't recommend using them daily. The original steps of cleansing followed separately by conditioning are still important and shouldn't be discarded based on expediency alone. I myself use a one-step product every two or three days. This particular formula is easy to make and smells tropical and exotic. Your hair will be clean and full of shine, with just the right amount of conditioning.

For All Hair Types

Purpose: To add a natural conditioner to your favorite shampoo.

Remember to do your patch test (page xiii).

shampoo: cleanser
coconut milk: strengthener
macadamia nut oil: conditioner
canola oil: conditioner
mayonnaise: conditioner

Botanical Formula

$^1/_4$ cup shampoo*

1 teaspoon coconut milk

1 teaspoon macadamia nut oil

1 teaspoon canola oil

1 tablespoon mayonnaise

In a blender, mix all ingredients together on low speed for 20 to 30 seconds, or until smooth. Wet hair with warm water and massage shampoo into hair, lathering well. Rinse with warm water.

SHELF LIFE: Cover and refrigerate; discard after 3 days.

---

*Commercial shampoo should not be a one-step shampoo (with conditioner), a dandruff shampoo, or an oily hair shampoo.

Beer and Egg
Shampoo Enhancer

For Normal to Dry Hair

Purpose: To add strength, shine, softness, and manageability to your hair by enhancing your favorite shampoo.

Remember to do your patch test (page xiii).

shampoo: cleanser
beer: softener
egg: softener
lemon extract: shine
orange extract: softener; shine
banana extract: softener; shine

If you happen to live in an area with hard water, your hair most likely suffers from lack of softness and shine. The buildup of calcium and magnesium ions in the water affects the cleansing and rinsing action of shampoos, resulting in dull, lifeless hair.

Use this formula as needed, even daily. If your water is soft and you still suffer from lack of body and bounce, this formula will help your hair and keep it smelling great.

Botanical Formula

$^1/_4$ cup shampoo

1 teaspoon beer (nonlight beer)

1 egg

1 teaspoon lemon extract

$^1/_4$ teaspoon orange extract

$^1/_4$ teaspoon banana extract

Mix all ingredients together in a small bowl until smooth. Mixture may foam up a bit. Wet hair with warm water, massage shampoo into hair, lathering well, then rinse with warm water. Makes $^1/_4$ cup.

SHELF LIFE: Cover and refrigerate; discard after 2 days.

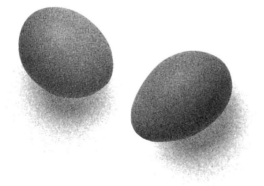

Clove and Apple Dandruff Shampoo

If you suffer from dandruff, try this recipe as a fun and effective alternative to your current product. It exfoliates dead skin cells from the scalp and removes buildup of oil and hair care products. The clove adds a natural zest to this recipe. Grown from the evergreen clove tree, this distinctive little spice has been used medicinally for soothing body pain to toothaches. In this recipe, they medicate and soothe the scalp during this process, leaving your head feeling tingly and stimulated.

This formula should be used at least three times a week for normal dandruff sufferers. If your dandruff is caused by an allergy, however, do not expect a dramatic result. The ingredients are designed only to address normal dryness and irritation.

For All Hair Types

Purpose: To reduce or significantly diminish dandruff after one week of treatment.

Remember to do your patch test (page xiii).

shampoo: cleanser
apple cider vinegar: dandruff reducer
apple juice: dandruff reducer
rum extract: buildup remover
cloves: antiseptic; anesthetic

Botanical Formula

$^1/_4$ *cup shampoo**

1 tablespoon apple cider vinegar

3 tablespoons apple juice

$^1/_2$ *teaspoon rum extract*

6 finely ground cloves

In a blender, mix all ingredients together on low speed for 30 to 40 seconds, or until completely mixed. Small bits of clove will remain evident in the solution. Shampoo as usual, scrubbing scalp thoroughly, and rinse thoroughly with warm water. Makes $^1/_4$ cup.

SHELF LIFE: Cover and refrigerate; discard after 3 days.

---

*Commercial shampoo should not be a one-step shampoo (with conditioner), a dandruff shampoo, or an oily hair shampoo.

Apple Cider Dandruff Flake Removal Shampoo

For All Hair Types

Purpose: To remove dead skin or flakes from scalp and hair.

Remember to do your patch test (page xiii).

apple cider vinegar: exfoliant

lemon extract: exfoliant; softener

egg yolks: softener

The physical evidence of dandruff is the small flakes that collect on the surface of our scalp and eventually find their way down to our shoulders. Use this formula to remove the existing flakes and dead skin forming on the scalp. Both lemons and apple cider vinegar are great exfoliators of dead skin cells.

This shampoo is followed by a rinse that accentuates the removal of flaking with an added dose of apple cider vinegar that remains in the hair to some degree even after rinsing. This is a great daily treatment for dandruff-afflicted scalps. I recommend using the Preventative Dandruff Treatment (see next formula) once a week to complement and enhance the effects of this shampoo and rinse.

Botanical Formula

SHAMPOO:

1 tablespoon apple cider vinegar

1 tablespoon lemon extract

3 egg yolks

$1/_2$ cup warm water

RINSE:

1 cup warm water

1 tablespoon apple cider vinegar

In a blender, mix shampoo ingredients together on low speed for 20 seconds. In a separate container, whisk the rinse ingredients together for 10 seconds. Massage shampoo into the hair and leave on for 10 minutes. For rinse, combine rinse ingredients in a cup and pour over hair after shampooing, followed by warm water and a conditioner. Makes $3/4$ cup shampoo, 1 cup rinse.

SHELF LIFE:Cover and refrigerate; discard after 3 days.

Oregano Hair Detangler

Oregano possesses the amazing ability to detangle hair and add manageability that hair loses if it's overworked or overmanaged. Since oregano has such a distinctive aroma, the addition of vanilla as a scent creates a warm, sweet fragrance for the hair. The vanilla also adds shine and luster.

Botanical Formula

$^1/_2$ cup fresh oregano leaves

1 teaspoon pure vanilla extract

1 cup water

In a small saucepan, heat all ingredients together on low. Let simmer for 30 minutes. Remove from heat and strain mixture, filtering out particles. When solution cools, pour into a spray bottle. After shampooing and conditioning, spray solution directly onto hair, saturating strands and scalp. Comb through immediately and leave on. Makes $^1/_2$ cup.

SHELF LIFE: Refrigerate in spray bottle; discard after 3 days.

For All Hair Types

Purpose: To assist in combing through tangled hair and to increase manageability.

Remember to do your patch test (page xiii).

oregano: detangler; softener
vanilla extract: scent

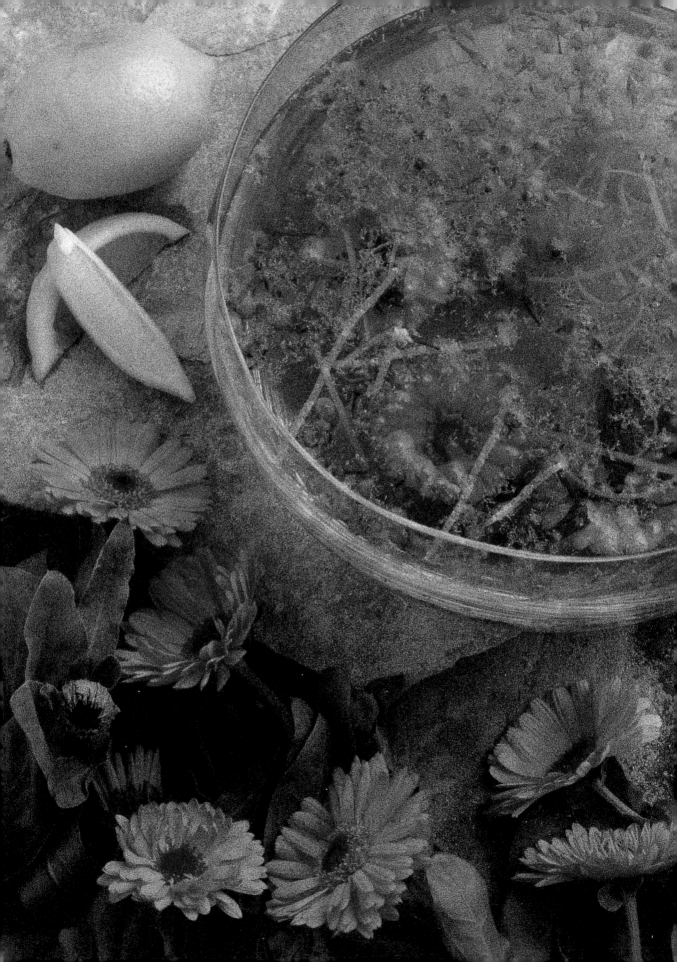

Chamomile and Calendula Hair Lightener

Sunshine for the hair, that's chamomile and calendula. These brightly colored flowers even resemble the sun. This recipe softly lightens and brightens fair hair, blonde to light brown, leaving it soft and supple. Gentle, playful highlights burst forth, adding texture and depth of color. Using this rinse every other day will ensure a consistent lightness and softness to your hair. As a natural rinse, it is not meant to be permanent.

For All Hair Types

Purpose: To lighten and brighten blonde hair with a temporary rinse.

Remember to do your patch test (page xiii).

chamomile flowers: lightener
calendula flowers: lightener
lemon juice: shine; C
lemon extract: shine; softener

Botanical Formula

4 cups water

2 cups dried chamomile flowers

2 cups dried calendula flowers (pot marigold)

1 tablespoon lemon juice

1 tablespoon lemon extract

In a saucepan, bring water, chamomile, and calendula to a boil. Reduce heat, cover, and simmer for 45 minutes. Remove from heat and cool, stirring in lemon juice and extract. When cooled enough for application, massage into hair, making sure that concentrated amounts stay in hair, and cover with plastic. Leave on for at least 40 minutes, then rinse with warm water. Use every other day for lasting effects. Makes 4 cups.

SHELF LIFE: Cover and refrigerate; discard after 5 days.

Cherry-Almond Hair Mist

For Normal to Dry Hair

Purpose: To moisten and softens dry hair and add shine.

Remember to do your patch test (page xiii).

almond extract: softener; scent

cherry extract: softener; scent

vanilla extract: softener; scent

lemon juice: shine; C

Hair, like the body, needs an occasional lift. It gets tired and loses its shine and bounce. A hair mist is great because it's designed to be left on the hair after shampooing and conditioning. Sprayed on while hair is still wet, it penetrates the shaft, sealing in moisture and giving a rich luster and shine. This delicious combination of softening agents, or laminates—almond, cherry, and vanilla—gives hair back the silky softness it once had.

Botanical Formula

1 teaspoon almond extract

1 teaspoon cherry extract

1 teaspoon vanilla extract

4 teaspoons lemon juice

2 cups water

Mix all ingredients together in a spray bottle. Shake well and then apply by spraying onto hair. Massage into hair with fingers or comb. Makes 2$\frac{1}{8}$ cups.

SHELF LIFE: Refrigerate; discard after 1 week.

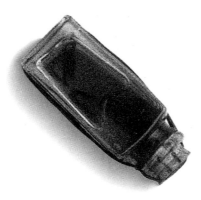

Black Tea–Rosemary Rinse for Dark Brown Hair

The robust, intense qualities of black teas and richly roasted coffees that turn on our bodies, now turn on our hair. Using coffee and tea to enhance and tone your natural deep brown hair seems like an obvious choice. Their inherent permeability, which we know as stains, is the perfect attribute for coloring brown hair. Rosemary is also an exceptional coloring agent for brown hair. It has been used for thousands of years as a color rinse to enhance and balance brown tones and to condition hair.

This recipe can be used on light to dark brown hair and will darken the lighter shades. For less intensity, try using 1 teaspoon less coffee and 1 less tea bag. Also, this recipe is designed to gradually wash out with frequent shampooing. If you want to maintain a darker color, use this rinse every day or every other day.

A Natural Hair Coloring

Purpose: To add natural dark brown highlights and color hair without harsh and damaging chemicals.

Remember to do your patch test (page xiii).

black tea: color agent
oregano leaves: color agent
rosemary leaves: color agent
coffee: color agent
lemon extract: shine; softener

Botanical Formula

7 bags black tea or 2¹/₂ tablespoons loose tea

2 tablespoons chopped oregano leaves

2 tablespoons chopped rosemary leaves

2 cups water

1 tablespoon instant coffee

1 tablespoon lemon extract

In a saucepan over medium heat, mix the tea, oregano, and rosemary with the water; steep for 45 to 50 minutes. Remove tea bags and filter out oregano, rosemary, and loose tea if used. Liquid may be placed into a small pitcher. Add coffee and lemon extract to liquid, and stir until combined. Let cool and then slowly pour solution over your head, a little at a time, massaging into hair and scalp, covering all strands thoroughly. This should be done standing in your bathtub, as the solution has a very thin consistency. Let sit for 30 minutes, covered with plastic, until it dries slightly. Rinse with warm water. Makes 1¹/₂ cups.

SHELF LIFE: Cover and refrigerate; discard after 5 days.

Citrus Hair Lightener

For All Hair Types

Purpose: To naturally lighten hair.

Remember to do your patch test (page xiii).

lemon juice: lightener; C
lime juice: lightener; C
lemon extract: lightener; softener
lime extract: lightener; softener

If you have fair hair, you no doubt love the effect the sun has on it, making it brighter and lighter. How do you achieve that lightening effect quickly and effectively? Lemons and limes, of course. They act with the sunlight to quickly lighten and brighten fair hair, adding shine and shimmer.

This lightener is easy to make and easy to apply. I recommend applying it a couple of times during a sunning period, and following it with a moisturizing oil treatment.

Botanical Formula

2 tablespoons fresh lemon juice

2 tablespoons fresh lime juice

1 tablespoon lemon extract

1 teaspoon lime extract

In a spray bottle, mix all of the ingredients. Shake bottle and spray all over hair. Massage into hair shafts and scalp. Go directly outside and remain in sunlight for at least 30 minutes. Apply several times a day while outside. This application tends to dry hair, so always follow with a moisturizing oil treatment. Makes 1/4 cup.

WARNING: Keep solution away from eyes.

SHELF LIFE: Refrigerate in bottle immediately; discard after 1 week.

Chocolate-Pumpkin Conditioning Hair Milk

Hair will luxuriate happily in this rich, great-smelling conditioning milk. It restores moisture and shine to hair, makes it soft to the touch, and adds volume and bounce to tired strands. The whole formula is scented deliciously with chocolate and vanilla.

Botanical Formula

1 tablespoon vegetable oil

1 tablespoon coconut oil

2 tablespoons chopped pumpkin

2 tablespoons coconut milk

1 teaspoon almond extract

1 teaspoon chocolate extract

1 teaspoon vanilla extract

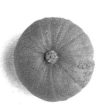

For Normal to Dry Hair

Purpose: To periodically treat hair with extra moisture, softness, and volume.

Remember to do your patch test (page xiii).

vegetable oil: softener
coconut oil: softener
pumpkin: moisturizer; A
coconut milk: volumizer
almond extract: shine enhancer
chocolate extract: scent
vanilla extract: scent

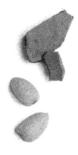

In a small saucepan, heat vegetable and coconut oils until slightly warm, mixing together. Remove and cool. Add remaining ingredients to oils and mix in blender until uniform. Massage mixture through hair and comb through carefully. Leave on for 5 minutes, then rinse thoroughly with warm water. Massage vigorously to remove all of the mixture, and continue rinsing until gone. Formula does not need to be reheated for subsequent applications; however, it does need to be stirred to ensure uniformity. May be used twice a week. Makes ¹/₂ cup.

SHELF LIFE: Cover and refrigerate; discard after 5 days.

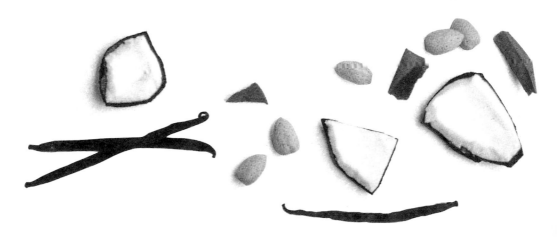

Cherry-Almond
Shampoo Additive

For All Hair Types

*Purpose: To strengthen
and add volume to hair
during shampooing.*

*Remember to do your
patch test (page xiii).*

shampoo: cleanser
egg: softener; volumizer
**maple syrup: strengthener;
volumizer**
vanilla extract: softener
almond extract: softener
cherry extract: softener

Immerse yourself in this sweet, fragrant volumizer, and emerge with a fabulously soft head of hair. During the cleansing process, your hair will receive a boost from maple syrup and egg. Deliciously scented with rich cherry nougat, it will bounce with restored health and luxurious shine.

Botanical Formula

1 cup shampoo*

1 whole egg

1 tablespoon real maple syrup

1 teaspoon vanilla extract

1 teaspoon almond extract

1 teaspoon cherry extract

In a blender, combine all ingredients on low speed for 40 seconds. Wet hair with warm water and massage shampoo into hair, lathering well. Rinse with warm water.

SHELF LIFE: Cover and refrigerate; discard after 3 days.

---

*Commercial shampoo should not be a one-step shampoo (with conditioner), a dandruff shampoo, or an oil hair shampoo.

Avocado
Hair Conditioner

Avocado oil penetrates the hair and scalp in this intensive, all-purpose hair conditioner. It nourishes the skin, hydrating the hair follicle and moisturizing the hair shaft, restoring luster and shine. Coconut oil lightly scents this moisturizing conditioner, which should be used every few days.

For Dry Brittle Hair

Purpose: To condition the hair, leaving it soft, manageable, and shiny.

Remember to do your patch test (page xiii).

Botanical Formula

2 teaspoons avocado oil

2 tablespoons olive oil

2 teaspoons canola oil

2 tablespoons vegetable shortening

2 teaspoons coconut oil*

2 teaspoons honey

avocado oil: conditioner
olive oil: conditioner
canola oil: conditioner
vegetable shortening: conditioner
coconut oil: scent
honey: softener

In a small saucepan, slowly warm all ingredients except honey over low heat. Remove from heat and cool. Add honey and stir in until mixed. Massage mixture through hair with fingers, comb through, and leave on for up to 20 minutes. Rinse with warm water. Makes 1/2 cup.

SHELF LIFE: Cover and refrigerate; discard after 5 days.

---

* If coconut oil is not available, use an extract. Add extract to mixture at same time as honey.

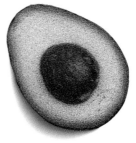

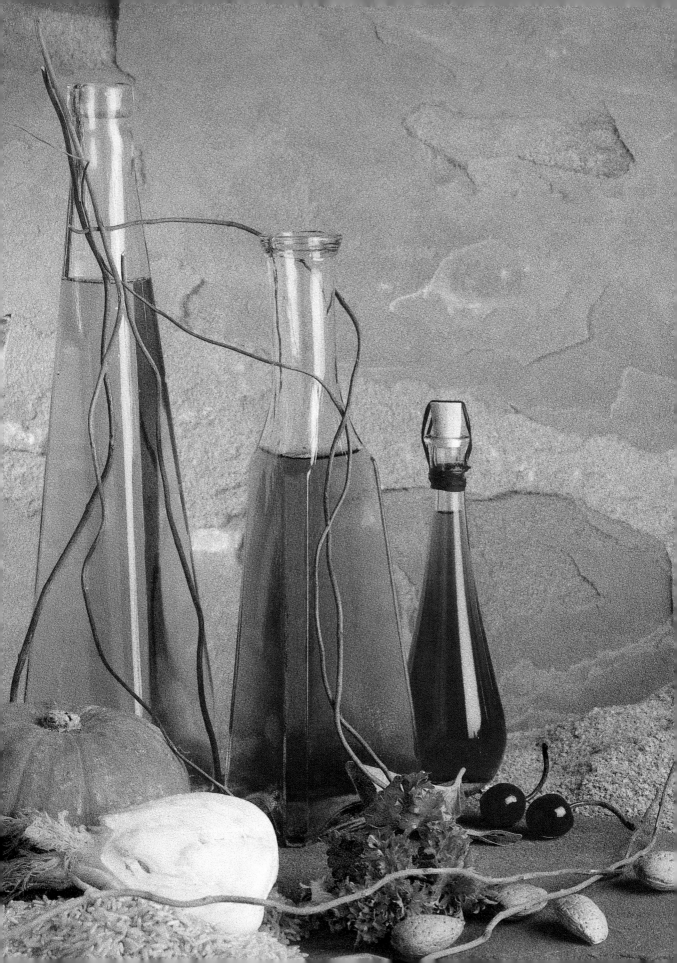

Special Remedies & Warm Weather Treatments

Special Remedies & Warm Weather Treatments

TIRED, ACHING FEET; DRY, CHAPPED HANDS; skin plagued by psoriasis or eczema…these are the problems addressed in this chapter. Give your feet a special treat by blending mint and mustard with lemon, cucumber, and water for a soothing foot soak, then massaging your feet with a mixture of cinnamon oil, peppermint, pineapple, and rosemary. Blend hazelnut and other oils with citrus extracts to make a moisturizer for dry, damaged hands. Soothe skin plagued by psoriasis or eczema with a cooling treatment made of anise, basil, parsley, and black tea, all of which possess healing and soothing properties.

Most of us have suffered from sunburn and have longed for a treatment that would relieve the burning, itching, and blistering of burned skin. This chapter devotes an entire section to warm-weather treatments, including a soothing bath formula containing oatmeal and rosemary, a blister treatment of black tea and salt, and a treatment that features oolong tea, cucumber, and lemon extract to help reduce sunburn pain and irritation. Finally, if mosquitoes are a problem in your area, be sure to try the simple Mosquito Bite Relief Pack next time you or someone you know is bitten.

Wrinkles should merely indicate where smiles have been.

—MARK TWAIN

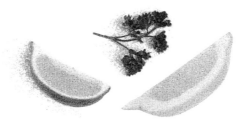

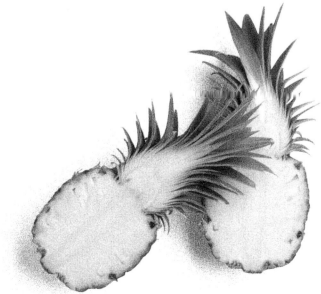

Minty Mustard Foot and Ankle Soak

Purpose: To soothe tense, tight, tired feet and ankles and reduce swelling.

Remember to do your patch test (page xiii).

cucumber: refresher
lemon: astringent; soother; C
mint: refresher
mustard: anti-inflammatory
lemon extract: softener
peppermint extract: stimulant

I recently met a farmer in Santa Fe, New Mexico, who grows the most amazing mustard. It has a powerfully spicy aroma and is incredibly flavorful. Munching on a few leaves at a time, I can feel the enzymes of this zesty cabbage working away, sending off warm, exotic firecrackers in my mouth.

A natural, healing soak with mustard is the perfect cure-all for all of the symptoms of overworked feet. The mustard, whether fresh or powdered, reduces swelling and soreness, going deep into afflicted tissue and bringing it relief. Your feet will thank you for this treat. I recommend using this soak as often as possible. For an additional treat, use a washcloth during the soak to rub and invigorate feet even more.

Botanical Formula

$1/4$ cucumber (chopped, do not peel)

$1/2$ lemon (peeled, seeded)

4 gallons water

1 cup chopped fresh mint

$1/8$ teaspoon mustard powder or
3 mustard leaves

1 teaspoon lemon extract

$1/4$ cup peppermint extract

In a blender, mix cucumber and lemon on medium speed until smooth. In a large pot, heat water until boiling and add mint. Remove from heat and let sit until temperature becomes manageable for your feet to soak in. Transfer to a plastic bucket or container large enough to hold mixture. Make sure that water level is high enough to cover ankles. Add cucumber, lemon, mustard, and extracts and stir. Soak feet and ankles for 15 minutes, or until water cools.

SHELF LIFE: Discard after 1 use.

Rosemary Milk Tonic for Feet

At the end of a hard day or night, treat yourself to this invigorating and soothing tonic that lifts the spirits as it tingles and teases your tired feet. Warm milk washed over your aching muscles, bringing soothing relief and softening of the skin. Your feet will feel so good that you'll want to use this every day.

Purpose: To soothe and relax tired feet.

Remember to do your patch test (page xiii).

milk: soother; A, D
mint: stimulant
rosemary: stimulant
peppermint extract: conditioner

Botanical Formula

1 cup hot milk

¹/₂ cup mint leaves

6 stems and leaves of rosemary

2 teaspoons peppermint extract

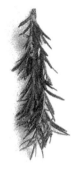

In a saucepan, simmer milk, mint, and rosemary over low heat for 15 minutes. Remove from heat and let cool slightly. Strain mixture through a filter, and stir in peppermint extract. Soak a clean, dry cloth with mixture and apply to feet, wrapping material around feet. Wrap in plastic if necessary. May be applied with a cotton ball instead for lighter treatment. Makes ¹/₂ cup, enough for 1 application.

SHELF LIFE: Discard after using.

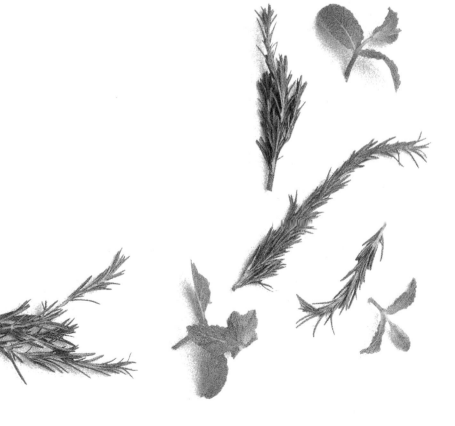

Pineapple-Anise Foot Smoother

Purpose: To remove rough skin from feet, stimulate circulation, and reduce pain in the feet.

Remember to do your patch test (page xiii).

pineapple: exfoliant; bromelain; A, C

apple: malic acid; A, C

lemon: exfoliant; astringent; C

grapefruit: exfoliant; astringent; citric acid; C

cinnamon oil: antiseptic; stimulant

mint leaves: stimulant

buttermilk: exfoliant; cleanser; lactic acid

anise: soother; healant

salt: soother

We often neglect our poor feet. They absorb our weight all day long and carry us wherever we go. All of this activity takes its toll, resulting in toughened, hardened skin, especially on the soles and toes. Dry areas may appear, giving an overall rough feeling. To eliminate these problems, I recommend this exfoliating pack at least once a week, twice a week if you are on your feet most of the day.

Botanical Formula

$^1/_2$ cup chopped pineapple flesh

1 apple (cored and chopped, do not peel)

$^1/_2$ lemon (peeled, seeded)

$^1/_8$ grapefruit (peeled, seeded)

1 teaspoon cinnamon oil*

1 teaspoon mint leaves

$^1/_4$ cup buttermilk

$^1/_2$ cup chopped anise bulb or 2 teaspoons anise extract

1 teaspoon salt

In a blender, mix all ingredients together on medium-low speed for 2 minutes, or until smooth. Rub mixture onto the feet, concentrating on the bottom of each foot and each heel. Wrap feet in plastic and leave on for 15 to 20 minutes. Rinse with warm water.

SHELF LIFE: Cover and refrigerate immediately; discard after 3 days.

*Cinnamon may irritate sensitive skin; omit from recipe if skin becomes red or irritated.

Luscious Lip Balm

Both men and women should apply lip balm daily to lips in order to maximize their sensually soft potential. What I love about this balm is that you customize it yourself, depending on your mood and personality.

I recommend certain flavored oils and extracts in this recipe because they are fairly easy to find. They are also fairly mild and won't overpower other scents you may have on your body. Other oils and extracts to try are coconut, strawberry, lemon, almond, anise, cherry, vanilla, and peppermint. Or if you have a particular flavor that you like, by all means try it.

Botanical Formula

1 teaspoon olive oil

1 teaspoon canola oil

2 teaspoons honey

$^1/_4$ teaspoon cinnamon oil or extract (optional)*

1 teaspoon orange oil or extract (optional)*

In a small mixing bowl, stir together all ingredients until thoroughly combined. If you use coconut oil, you will need to heat it and the other ingredients together in order for the coconut oil to melt and disperse. Otherwise, heating is not necessary. Apply to the lips continually after absorption. Use daily. Makes 2 tablespoons.

SHELF LIFE: Store unrefrigerated; discard after 5 days.

---

*If you use extracts, which are water based, instead of flavored oils, the mixture will need to be shaken before each use.

Purpose: To treat dry, chapped lips.

Remember to do your patch test (page xiii).

olive oil: softener; emollient
canola oil: softener; emollient
honey: conditioner
cinnamon oil: emollient; scent
orange oil: emollient; scent

Pumpkin Pilaf Hand-Softening Pack

Purpose: To soften dry or damaged hands.

Remember to do your patch test (page xiii).

brown rice: soother; fiber; B, E; calcium; iron
cucumber: refresher
pumpkin: moisturizer; A
coconut milk: softener

In this formula, pumpkin gives rich, intensive healing to dry, damaged hands. Cold, brisk winds may have chapped your hands, or perhaps you're not moisturizing as often as you should. The symptoms are the same, and will disappear after you spread on this sweet-smelling, luxurious hand treatment. Your hands will feel invigorated and softened and look younger and stronger.

Botanical Formula

$^1/_2$ *cup brown rice*

1 *cup warm water*

$^1/_2$ *chopped cucumber (do not peel)*

$^1/_4$ *cup pumpkin (fresh or canned)*

2 *tablespoons coconut milk*

In a bowl, combine rice and warm water, stirring together; let sit for 1 hour. Filter rice and water through a coffee filter or paper towel, saving the water and discarding the rice solids. In a blender, mix the cucumber, pumpkin, and coconut milk together on medium speed for 30 seconds. Add rice water to the blender and mix on medium speed for another 15 seconds. Apply mixture all over hands, and cover with plastic wrap or gloves. Let sit for 15 minutes. Remove covering and rinse with warm water. Makes 2 cups.

SHELF LIFE: Cover and refrigerate immediately; discard after 4 days.

Hazelnut Moisturizer for Dry Hands

This rich, luxurious mixture of oils penetrates deep down into dry, damaged hands, moisturizing and rehydrating dry skin cells and tissue. It quickly improves the look and feel of rough, chapped hands and, with daily use, will heal and protect hands from damaging elements in the environment.

Botanical Formula

1 tablespoon hazelnut oil*

1 teaspoon coconut oil or extract

1 tablespoon wheat germ oil*

1 teaspoon olive oil

1 teaspoon canola oil

1 tablespoon sesame oil

2 teaspoons lime extract

1 teaspoon lemon extract

Slowly heat oils together enough to melt the coconut oil. In a small bowl, combine warm oils and extracts and whisk vigorously for 30 seconds, or until homogeneous. Smooth product all over hands until completely covered. Wipe off any excess product. For every subsequent use, microwave until slightly warm, shake to mix, and apply as usual. There will be a slight separation between oils and water-based extracts. For dry hands, use daily. Makes $1/2$ cup.

SHELF LIFE: Store at room temperature away from heat source such as a stove. Discard after 1 week.

*If hazelnut oil is unavailable, use macadamia nut oil. If wheat germ oil is unavailable, use rice bran oil. Try health food stores for all four.

Purpose: To treat hands dried out by environmental or external conditions. Moisturizes normal skin to prevent drying.

Remember to do your patch test (page xiii).

hazelnut oil: moisturizer

coconut oil: moisturizer; scent

wheat germ oil: nutrient; moisturizer

olive oil: moisturizer

canola oil: moisturizer

sesame oil: moisturizer; emollient

lime extract: emollient

lemon extract: emollient

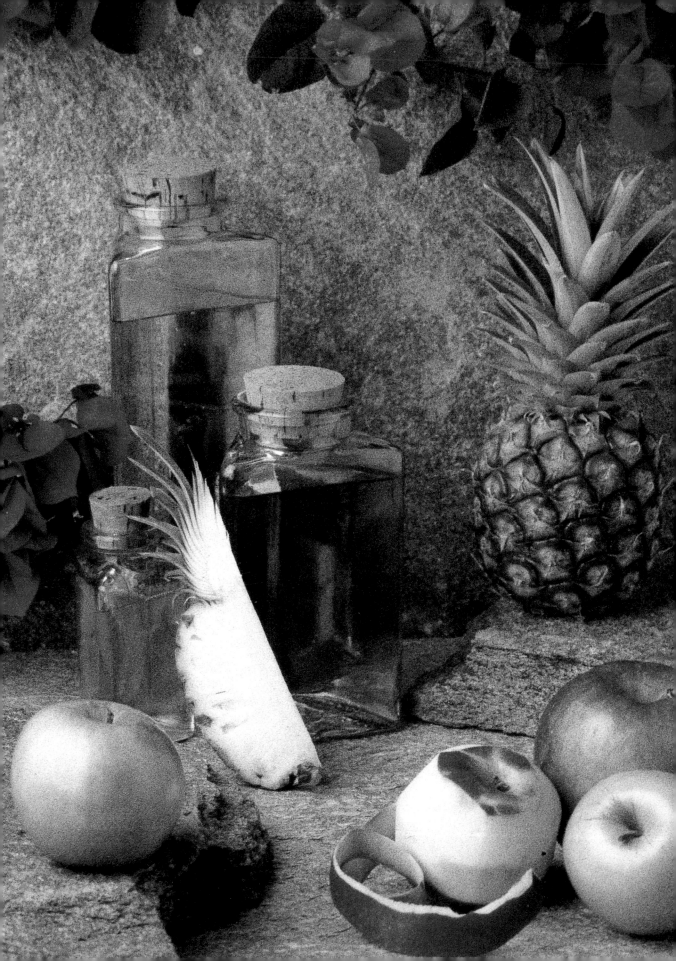

Pineapple-Honey Nail and Cuticle Treatment

The pineapple in this formula helps soften the cuticles, making them easier to trim or push back. This treatment should be applied at least once a week, if not more often, depending on how much abuse your hands take. If you live in a cold climate, you may want to use it more, to counteract the drying, chapping effects of wind and cold temperatures. Maintaining your nail and cuticle area on a regular basis will guarantee better-looking nails and a long life for them as well.

Purpose: To soften cuticles and nails to avoid breakage, and to help in easing the cuticle back. To reduce inflammation around cuticle.

Remember to do your patch test (page xiii).

pineapple: exfoliant; anti-inflammatory; A, C; bromelain
apple cider vinegar: exfoliant
canola oil: moisturizer
honey: humectant
egg yolk: ingredient binder; softener

Botanical Formula

¹/₄ cup pineapple flesh

¹/₄ teaspoon apple cider vinegar

2 teaspoons canola oil

2 teaspoons honey

1 egg yolk

Blend all ingredients together on medium speed for 15 seconds. The canola oil has a tendency to separate rapidly from the other ingredients, so apply quickly. Rub mixture onto hands, concentrating on the nail and cuticle areas. Place hands in plastic gloves and leave on for 10 to 15 minutes. Remove gloves and rinse hands with warm water. Be sure to remix solution before each application. Use daily if needed. Makes ¹/₂ cup.

SHELF LIFE: Cover and refrigerate; discard after 3 days.

Lemon-Anise Exfoliating Rub
for Dry, Scaly Hands

Purpose: To remove dry, scaly skin from hands, leaving them soft and smooth.

Remember to do your patch test (page xiii).

lemon: exfoliant; C
lime: exfoliant; C
apple juice: exfoliant
anise: soother; healant
wheat germ: moisturizer; E
tarragon: invigorator
lemon extract: softener
egg: ingredient binder

Like any other part of the body, hands feel dry and scaly from time to time. When this happens, it is essential to apply first aid to your hands to remove the dead skin cells and condition the skin so your hands will look and feel better quickly. Follow this treatment with a rich moisturizer to give extra hydration, if needed.

Botanical Formula

$1/2$ *lemon (peeled, seeded)*

$1/2$ *lime (peeled, seeded)*

$1/4$ *cup apple juice*

$1/2$ *cup chopped anise bulb or 2 teaspoons anise extract*

$1/4$ *cup wheat germ*

1 stem tarragon (with leaves, chopped)

1 teaspoon lemon extract

1 whole egg

In a blender, mix all ingredients together on low speed for 30 seconds. When completely blended, rub mixture on hands. Leave on for 10 to 15 minutes. If desired, wrap in plastic wrap or in gloves. Rinse with warm water. Makes $3/4$ cup.

SHELF LIFE: Cover and refrigerate; discard after 5 days.

Cinnamon-Pineapple
Foot Rub with Mint

Cinnamon has a naturally invigorating warmth about it that makes it ideal for a foot rub. Once valued in the West because of its scarcity, it is now a common spice harvested from the bark of the cinnamon tree of Asia. Together with the mint leaves, it stimulates circulation, leaving feet feeling refreshed and tingly. Cinnamon also helps fight bacteria existing on the feet, which are more prone to bacterial infection.

After rinsing this foot rub away, your feet will feel more alive. Roughness will be reduced, and the soreness and aching associated with fatigue and overexertion will vanish.

Botanical Formula

1 teaspoon cinnamon oil

2 teaspoons chopped mint leaves

1/4 cup chopped pineapple flesh

1 teaspoon chopped basil

1/4 cup peppermint extract*

2 tablespoons rosemary

In a blender, mix all ingredients together on medium speed for 45 seconds, or until blended thoroughly. Rub mixture into feet (top and bottom) and wrap in plastic. Let sit for 5 to 10 minutes, no more than 20 minutes, remove plastic, and rinse feet with warm water. Makes 1/2 cup.

SHELF LIFE: Cover and refrigerate immediately; discard after 5 days.

*For less stimulation, reduce amount of peppermint extract by at least half.

Purpose: To reduce pain in feet caused by sore muscles; to reduce swelling, aches, and presence of bacteria.

Remember to do your patch test (page xiii).

cinnamon oil: invigorator; bactericide
mint leaves: stimulant
pineapple: anti-inflammatory; bromelain; A, C
basil: conditioner; stimulant
peppermint extract: stimulant
rosemary: stimulant; antiseptic

Cooling Psoriasis Relief Treatment

Purpose: To reduce scaliness and soften psoriasis-affected areas of skin.

Remember to do your patch test (page xiii).

anise bulb: soother
basil: soother
parsley: healant
black tea: healant

The dryness and scaliness associated with psoriasis can be painful and irritating. This annoying skin disorder, generally inherited, causes skin to develop at a faster rate than normal. The result is red skin layered with scaly, white clusters, usually on joints, such as knees and elbows, and often on the scalp, hands, or feet.

The cooling action from this treatment will bring instant relief from the itching and will reduce irritation and redness. Anise, an ancient member of the parsley family, is probably best known as the source of anise seeds, which lend a powerful licorice flavor to foods and liquors, such as anisette and ouzo. The clean, soothing properties of this plant cool and relieve rough, red skin. Using this treatment daily will not rid you of psoriasis, but it will make it far more tolerable.

Botanical Formula

1 anise bulb, cut into pieces

3 cups water

1 tablespoon basil

1 tablespoon parsley

1 cup steeped black tea

In a blender, mix anise on medium speed until smooth. In a small saucepan, heat water, basil, and parsley until boiling; then reduce heat and simmer for 45 minutes. Remove from heat and cool. Mix liquid with anise and tea in small mixing bowl. If you don't want herbs in the final mixture, filter them out before using liquid. Apply mixture with a clean cloth to psoriasis-affected areas every 30 minutes for 2 hours every night. Makes 2 cups.

SHELF LIFE: Cover and refrigerate; discard after 5 days.

Suntanning Soothing and Cleansing Mist

This cool, refreshing mist is easy to apply while sunbathing or doing any kind of activity outside, because it sprays on lightly, never feeling sticky or thick on the skin. A quick spritz of this mist on the body and face will help keep it clean no matter how long you are outside and no matter how much you are perspiring.

Botanical Formula

1 teaspoon hydrogen peroxide (2.5% active, or less)

1 teaspoon lemon extract

1 teaspoon cucumber extract (see page xiii)

1 cup water

Combine all ingredients together in a small spray bottle and shake for 10 seconds. Spray onto face and body periodically during sunbathing. Makes 1 cup.

WARNING: Avoid spraying solution in eyes.

SHELF LIFE: Refrigerate; discard after 4 days.

Purpose: To moisten and soothe the skin during sunbathing.

Remember to do your patch test (page xiii).

hydrogen peroxide: antiseptic

lemon extract: astringent; toner

cucumber extract: soother; toner

Coconut Tanning Oil

Purpose: To moisturize and lubricate the skin while attracting sun.

Remember to do your patch test (page xiii).

olive oil: lubricant
castor oil: lubricant
vegetable oil: lubricant
coconut oil: lubricant

This is a great, all-purpose, lubricating tanning oil, designed for medium to dark-toned skin types. Users should be warned, however, that overexposure to the sun does cause long-term damage to the skin, and using these oils intensifies the effects of the sun. A commercial sunblock would be a great complement to this recipe, as it would inhibit some of the damage from ultraviolet rays.

After your tanning session, rinse off in lukewarm water and slip into something slinky and small and savor your heightened skin tone.

Botanical Formula

$^1/_4$ cup olive oil

2 tablespoons castor oil

$^1/_4$ cup vegetable oil

$^1/_4$ teaspoon coconut oil

In a small saucepan, slowly warm all ingredients together, stirring in order to distribute the coconut oil, which tends to form solids. Remove from heat and allow to cool. Apply by spreading and massaging on skin before sunbathing. Makes approximately $^1/_2$ cup.

SHELF LIFE: Cover and refrigerate; discard after 1 week.

Black Tea
Sunburn Treatment Masque

Grapes are natural demulcents, bringing relief and healing to the skin. In this formula they help to reduce redness and inflammation due to sunburn. This creamy, smooth masque will coat the skin and provide first aid with soothing, healing relief.

Purpose: To soothe sun-burned areas of the body (shoulders, neck, legs).

Remember to do your patch test (page xiii).

black tea: healant
grapes: anti-inflammatory; soother; A, C; enzymes
cucumber: soother
baking soda: soother

Botanical Formula

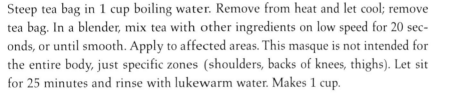

1 black tea bag

1 cup water

8 seedless grapes

$1/_2$ cucumber (do not peel)

1 teaspoon baking soda

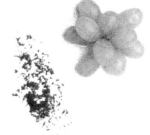

Steep tea bag in 1 cup boiling water. Remove from heat and let cool; remove tea bag. In a blender, mix tea with other ingredients on low speed for 20 seconds, or until smooth. Apply to affected areas. This masque is not intended for the entire body, just specific zones (shoulders, backs of knees, thighs). Let sit for 25 minutes and rinse with lukewarm water. Makes 1 cup.

SHELF LIFE: Cover and refrigerate immediately; discard after 4 days.

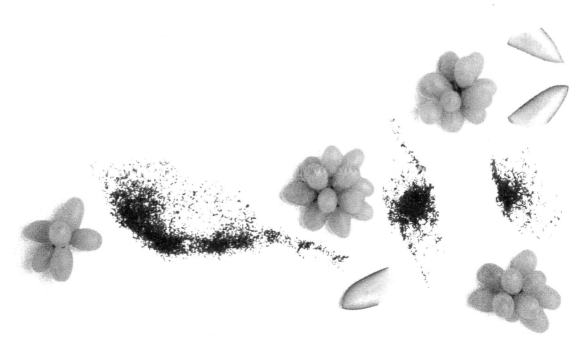

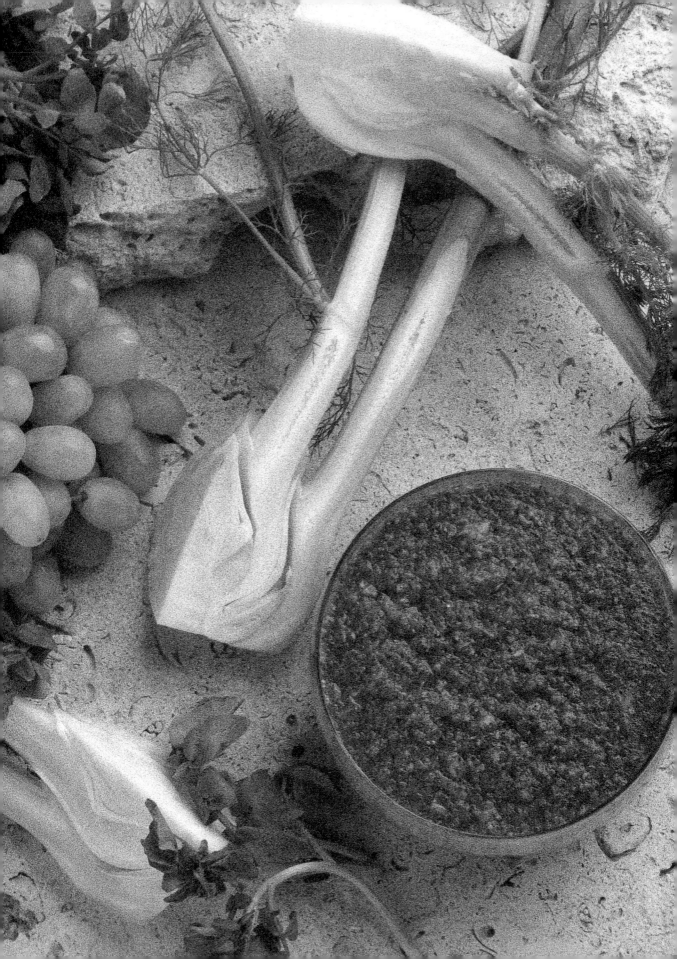

Soothing Eczema and Psoriasis Masque

Both eczema and psoriasis result in patchy, rough skin. If the symptoms are not treated, the result is dry, scaly skin that looks and feels old and tough. A gentle cleansing masque that also soothes and cools is a great treatment for the pain associated with these problems.

While this treatment will not cure you of your skin disorder, it will relieve the pain and discomfort. It also takes away some of the excess skin and flakiness associated with these disorders, leaving skin softer and smoother.

Botanical Formula

$^1/_4$ *chopped watercress*

10 white seedless grapes

2 tablespoons baking soda

1 anise stem

2 teaspoons anise extract

5 tablespoons water

In a blender, mix all ingredients together on medium speed for 30 seconds, or until smooth. Place mixture on affected areas and wrap in plastic wrap (optional). Leave on for 30 minutes. Rinse with warm water. Makes $^3/_4$ cup.

SHELF LIFE: Cover and refrigerate; discard after 3 days.

Purpose: To soothe and improve the appearance of areas affected by eczema and psoriasis.

Remember to do your patch test (page xiii).

watercress: medicant
grapes: anti-inflammatory; softener; A, C; enzymes
baking soda: cleanser; soother
anise stem: soother
anise extract: soother

Soothing Rosemary-Oatmeal Sunburn Bath

Purpose: To soothe sunburn pain during the first 24 to 48 hours after a sunburn.

Remember to do your patch test (page xiii).

cucumber: refresher
oatmeal: pain reliever; moisturizer; B, E
black tea: healant, soother
rosemary leaves: pain reliever

This is an extraordinary treatment for the entire body. Sunburn not only hurts, it also itches and tightens the skin. This rosemary bath will wash your body with soothing, calming effects, reducing overall body pain. The oatmeal relieves itching and irritation due to dryness, and the black tea, used in many sunburn treatments, helps cool the body and draw the heat away. I strongly recommend this bath at least once a day for the first few days after becoming sunburned.

Botanical Formula

1 cucumber

4 cups oatmeal

10 black tea bags

2 tablespoons rosemary leaves

Puree cucumber in a blender. In a mixing bowl, combine cucumber with all other ingredients and stir until mixed. Mixture will be slightly dry. With warm bath water running, empty mixture into water right under faucet. Let mixture disperse in water as bath fills. Stay in bath for up to 1 hour if possible. Use several times daily, as needed. Try to use immediately after being sunburned. Makes enough for 1 bath.

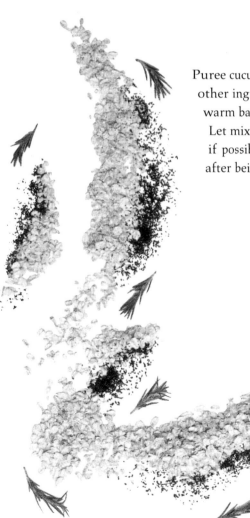

Sun Blister
Skin Treatment

Sunburn can be so painful. If you are unlucky enough to suffer from severe sunburn, resulting in blistering, try this treatment as soon as you come in from sunning. Black tea is ideal for soothing hot, sore skin. The salt helps fluid drain from the blisters. Skin will begin to peel by the next day, allowing new, undamaged skin to surface. The blistering and peeling will not look pretty, but at least they won't hurt as much.

Botanical Formula

2 black tea bags

3 cups water

1 tablespoon salt

Bring 2 cups water to a boil; remove from heat. Steep tea bags in water for 30 minutes, remove tea bags, and let cool. In a mixing bowl, stir tea together with salt and 1 cup water. Saturate a towel or cloth with solution and lay it flat onto the burned areas. Let sit for 15 to 25 minutes. Reapply as needed until skin is cooler and relieved of pain. Makes 3 cups.

SHELF LIFE: Discard after use.

Purpose: To treat sun-burned skin, removing blisters and starting the healing process in skin.

Remember to do your patch test (page xiii).

black tea: healant
salt: healant; soother

Lemony Oolong Tea Sunburn Treatment

Purpose: To soothe sunburn pain and reduce blistering.

Remember to do your patch test (page xiii).

oolong tea: soother
oats: soother; B, E
cucumber: refresher
lemon extract: refresher
white vinegar: soother

Once again, tea comes to the rescue of sunburn pain and swelling. Oolong, a fermented tea that is not as dark as black tea, soothes skin and brings consistent relief from pain and irritation due to sunburn.

This treatment helps the skin heal faster and feel better more quickly. To reduce the effects of sunburn, use it as often as you need to throughout the first 24 hours after overexposure to the sun. You may be surprised at how great you feel the next day.

Botanical Formula

$3^1/_2$ cups water

6 oolong tea bags

1 tablespoon quick rolled oats

$^1/_2$ cup chopped cucumber (do not peel)

1 teaspoon lemon extract

1 teaspoon white vinegar

Bring 3 cups of the water to a boil, and immerse all 6 oolong tea bags; remove from heat and let steep for $^1/_2$ hour; let cool and remove tea bags. In a small bowl, combine $^1/_2$ cup water with oatmeal and stir together until mixed; strain mixture through a paper towel, saving liquid and discarding oats. In a blender, mix 1 tablespoon of oatmeal liquid together with cucumber, extract, and vinegar on medium speed for 1 minute, or until pureed. Strain mixture through a paper towel, saving liquid. In a bowl, stir together strained liquid and liquid tea. Saturate a cloth or towel with solution and place it on sunburned areas for 15 minutes. Reapply if necessary after first application until skin begins to feel relief. To help reduce blistering, this treatment must be applied immediately after burning.

SHELF LIFE: Discard after use.

Mosquito Bite Relief Pack

A good friend of mine who grew up in the South swears that she has used a recipe similar to this one for years. It may be common in that region, but most people in other areas of the country don't know about this easy and effective method of reducing the pain and swelling of a mosquito bite. To soothe affected areas, apply this relief pack liberally. It brings instant relief.

Purpose: To soothe areas swollen and irritated by mosquito bites.

Remember to do your patch test (page xiii).

baking soda: soother
almond extract: emollient

Botanical Formula

3 tablespoons baking soda

$1/2$ teaspoon almond extract

6 tablespoons water

In a small mixing bowl, combine all ingredients together by stirring until a paste forms. Apply pack to affected areas and let sit for 15 to 20 minutes. Rinse with warm water and pat dry.

SHELF LIFE: Not necessary to refrigerate. Store covered; discard after 3 days.

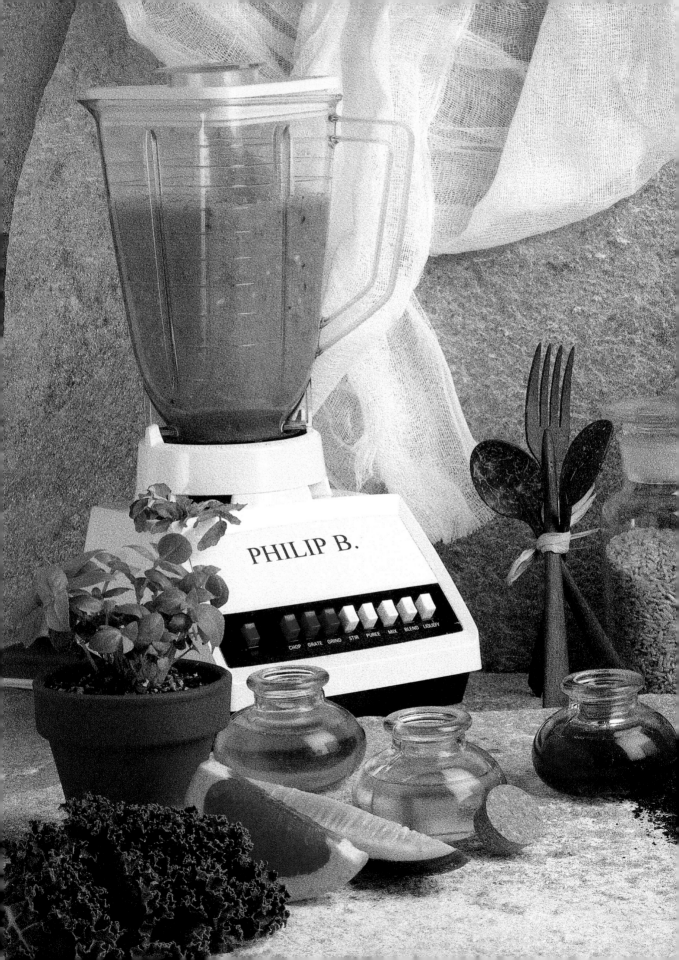

PHILIP B.

CHOP GRATE GRIND STIR PUREE MIX BLEND LIQUEFY

Appendices

Seasons of Change

HAVE YOU EVER NOTICED that your skin and hair resemble the current season? For instance, North American summers are generally hot and humid, producing an abundance of perspiration and secretion of oils from the body. Hair is moist but limp, whereas during cold weather, hair becomes dry and brittle, much like the barren landscape of winter. It is imperative to be aware of the changes in our bodies and to address these changes as they occur. It is even better to try to prevent the harsh changes as much as possible, thereby creating a year-long state of equilibrium for the skin and hair.

Spring

Spring is about renewal and rebirth. We shed our skin and awaken the mind and body from their wintry slumber. We stretch and reach up with the crocuses toward the warming sun. Small, delicate green leaves spring forth, signaling a new season, a rebirth of life. Soft, gentle breezes wash over us as we take in the sights and scents that welcome us into kinder, gentler conditions.

Spring is perhaps the kindest season of all when it comes to our bodies. Moisture levels in the air increase. The harsh winds of winter disappear, replaced by gentle breezes that caress instead of brutalize our skin. We begin spending more time outside in the sun. Our hair begins to reveal highlights, enhanced by the sun. Our skin begins to feel softer, less rough. To help it through this transition, it's important to exfoliate the old skin cells, in order to let the new layers, thriving during spring, be revealed. The Strawberry-Almond Facial Scrub is a wonderful seasonal treat for the face, exfoliating skin cells, lifting them away to reveal healthy skin underneath. The strawberry is one of the prizes of spring, so don't miss the opportunity to use this scrub to enhance your springtime skin. A great all-purpose cleanser is the Creamy Cucumber Facial Cleanser,

If truth is beauty, how come no one has their hair done in the library?

—LILY TOMLIN

which can also be used on the body. It's gentle enough for all skin types and gives cooling, soothing relief with a balance of astringency to fight oiliness.

The beginning of spring might be a good time for a new haircut, perhaps something shorter to help you move more easily into the warmer months. As the temperature begins to climb with the progression of the season, the body will begin producing more oils. A great body scrub to balance excess oil production is the Equatorial Enzyme Pack, for normal and dry skin types, which also provides moisture that may be lost during exfoliation. The Milky Soft Body Cleanser is a marvelous wash for all skin types, resulting in clean, soft skin with renewed tone. It helps even out any patchiness caused by dryness, diet, or bruising.

Hair will certainly be grateful for the warmer, moisture-rich days of spring, compared with the harshness of winter. To revitalize it after the cold months, try the Sesame-Coconut Protein Conditioner or Avocado Hair Conditioner, both designed to restore luster, shine, and manageability to moisture-starved, lackluster hair.

Summer

Summer is the season of frolicking and reveling in the glories of the sun. Hot, sweaty bodies litter the beaches and boardwalks. We pare down on clothing, revealing soft, supple tanned skin.

This freedom of exposure may be great for the psyche, but not for the skin. On the one hand, the intense moisture created during warmer weather is great for the skin. It hydrates and feeds the skin and releases us from the heavy moisturizing routines of winter. However, the drying and chapping effects of the sun and lengthy exposure to the elements outdoors can be devastating. The skin may look moist, but don't be fooled. Tiny wrinkles may begin to appear, the skin will take on a leathery feeling, and by the end of your glorious summer, you may start to feel like the dry leaves of fall.

Skin never gets any younger, so it's best to take care of it now. The skin is one of our most vital organs, not to mention the largest. Going from hot temperatures outdoors to cold, air-conditioned indoor environments subjects our bodies to climate shock, resulting in dehydrated, chapped skin.

Hair goes through similar abuse. It soaks in chlorine-filled pools and salty oceans and dries out from overexposure both to the sun and to cold, dry, air-conditioned environments such as houses, offices, and shopping malls. Some natural moisturizing is provided by the scalp, which produces an abundance of sebum during summer, offsetting some of the drying of the hair shaft, but it can also result in oily hair. Additional moisture is provided in the air, but if you live in an exceptionally humid area and you have slightly curly hair, you'll encounter an unwanted abundance of frizziness and lack of control.

Common sense can help you get through the summer. It's important to keep the skin clean and clear of excess dirt and sweat. Frequent cleansing and toners help balance the increased oil production of your body, especially on the face. The t-zone, or the area from your forehead down your nose and to your chin, is typically the problem area for most people during summer. Light, astringent toners, such as the Lemon-Lime Toner and Oil Remover, and the Cucumber-Parsley Facial Toner, help the skin start the day or end the night with a clear, healthy glow. The Facial Mist is a great all-day pickup for the face, providing a light and refreshing spritz to hot, tired skin. To help people with oily hair make it through this season, I recommend the Preshampooing Orange-Vodka Buildup Remover or the Vanilla-Rum Cocktail, both designed to lift off oils and dirt from the hair shaft and scalp, leaving them healthier and cleaner.

Fall

Fall has arrived, and with it we welcome the crisp nights filled with the crunching of old dead twigs under our feet and angels of red, yellow, and brown floating gently down around us as they fall from their perches. We reflect on the past and gather ourselves up for colder weather ahead. Fields are bursting with pumpkins, squash, and root vegetables. There is a sense of shutting down, of taking time to ponder the prior season and its vigor and life. Fall is a season rich with change. Warm, fuzzy sweaters and corduroy pants replace the light cottons and silks of summer.

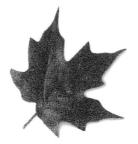

Skin goes through a phenomenal change when fall whisks around the corner. One morning we wake up and our skin isn't as smooth as it was yesterday. The winds are brisker and the air is cooler, drying the leaves outside as well as our skin and hair. The moisture that we both loved and hated during summer is gone, replaced by an increasingly arid climate. Days are now filled with kids going off to school, holiday planning, and a general increase in stress that takes a vicious toll on our bodies. Dry, flyaway strands of hair have lost their shine and bounce. Dry patches of skin begin appearing on our faces and bodies.

First aid is essential. The Indian Summer Body Pack is great for fighting overall body dryness. It soothes dry skin and replenishes moisture using two of fall's greatest finds, sweet potatoes and spaghetti squash. The Peach-Pumpkin Smoothie Conditioning Body Masque softens and hydrates skin, and the Pumpkin Power Deep Moisturizing Body Oil provides overnight deep penetration of oils, restoring suppleness and softness to skin. In between these intensive treatments, moisturize every day and night. You are waging a battle with the elements, so you have to take an aggressive course.

A seasonal treat for moisturizing hair is found in the Vegetarian Refried Bean Hair Masque, using, among other ingredients, sweet potatoes, which restore moisture to hair and provide vitamin A to the scalp. It is imperative to maintain proper moisture in the hair shaft and scalp. I recommend having a good haircut at the end of summer to eliminate split ends and help your hair start fresh with a new season. Moisture is vital during fall in order to maintain healthy shine and body. The Honey-Maple Hot Oil Treatment is a rich, oil-based treatment that penetrates the hair shaft and scalp and creates a seal around the shaft in order to maintain moisture balance.

> *The body is a sacred garment.*
>
> —MARTHA GRAHAM

Winter

Winter has its own version of beauty bleakness. If you live in the Northeast, where I grew up, you are accustomed to heavy snows, bitter winds, icy streets, and the parched, dried-out feeling that covers your entire body. Arms and legs feel as rough as the cold, barren trees outside. On the West Coast, where those from other parts of the country think the sun never stops shining, rain and cooler temperatures accompany increased dryness and brittleness. Gray days overlap, becoming a long string of monotonous, monochromatic indicators of the season of hibernation. Our bodies really go into shock during winter. It is a natural process, though. In order to have renewal and life, physical dormancy is necessary as part of the eternal cycle. Without the complementary seasons, we would have no balance in our lives.

A few helpful hints may help you get through the winter unscathed by its effects. First, try to take cooler showers and baths. Exposing your skin to hot water and then going out in the windy, cold air will dry and chap skin. I love baths during the winter. They cloak the body in a sea of warmth and sweet scents. The Orange-Coconut Bath Oil and the Oatmeal, Rice, and Coconut Bath will both provide the body with softness and will seal in moisture, helping skin to maintain its even tone and glow. The Honey-Oatmeal Facial Masque is great because it gently lifts off dead skin cells and moisturizes new skin underneath. Its gentle formula, designed specifically for sensitive skin, can be used on any skin type and provides a great balance during especially brutal weather.

Hair experiences real trauma during winter as well. It goes through the same seesaw effect as it does in summer, plunged from hot environments into cold ones. Most people overheat their houses and cars, saturating themselves with dry heat, followed by exposure to blasts of cold, dry air outside. Moisture is drawn away from the scalp, leaving it dry and flaky. Hair becomes brittle, resulting in breakage and a flat color and texture. The Chocolate-Pumpkin Conditioning Hair Milk or the Honey-Maple Hot Oil Treatment are both terrific for restoring bounce, body, and shine to dehydrated hair.

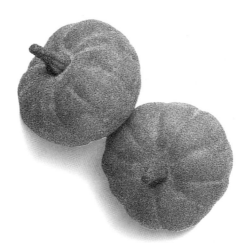

Conversion Chart

Dry

¼ cup = 4 tbs = 2 oz = 60g
1 cup = ½ pound = 8 oz = 250g

Liquid

¼ cup = 2 fl oz = 60 ml
1 cup = 8 fl oz = 250 ml

Miscellaneous

1 inch = 2.5 cm
zucchini = courgette
baking soda = bicarbonate of soda
rolled oats = oat flakes
skillet = frying pan

Glossary of Terms

Acid: A sour element that appears naturally in some foods, for example, malic acid in apples. Acids break down tissue, proteins, cell walls; used as an exfoliant.

Acorn squash: Used as a moisturizer in masques and scrubs; contains vitamin A; a winter squash with orange flesh and a hard, green shell.

Alfalfa sprouts: Soothes and treats skin; an astringent grown from germinated alfalfa seeds; low in calories; high in protein, minerals, and vitamins, especially vitamin C; sold fresh in supermarkets.

Almond: Exfoliant and scrub; skin lightener and emollient from the kernel of the fruit of the almond tree, grown in warm climates.

Amylase: Exfoliating enzyme found in apples.

Anesthetic: A drug that produces a lack of sensitivity to touch, temperature, and pain.

Anise: Medicant and soother; pore cleanser; soother of symptoms of eczema, psoriasis, and general irritation of the skin; member of carrot family containing aromatic seeds and flesh with a licorice flavor; if unavailable, use extract.

Anti-inflammatory: A substance that reduces inflammation and swelling of skin and tissue; reduces irritation.

Antiseptic: A substance that stops or inhibits the growth of bacteria.

Apple: An exfoliant used in masques and scrubs; contains malic acid, a protein digester; contains small amounts A and C. Apple seeds contain toxins; always be sure to remove the seeds in recipes which include apples.

Apple juice, apple cider vinegar: Help control dandruff flaking, remove excess oil, and provide astringency.

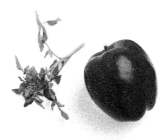

Apricot: Softener and emollient; oil remover and pore cleanser. Perishable fruit, cousin to the peach, soft yellow flesh with fuzzy, pale yellow exterior; contains vitamin A.

Artichoke: Skin conditioner; contains potassium and vitamin A. If using canned hearts, buy ones packed in water, not marinated in oil; member of the thistle family.

Astringent: A tightener and toner for the skin; temporarily reduces the size of pores; skin healer, refresher, invigorator, perspiration reducer.

Avocado: Moisturizer, emollient, skin, hair, and scalp conditioner used in masques and scrubs; fat-rich tropical fruit with buttery texture and mild flavor; high in unsaturated fat; contains vitamins A, C, D, and E, potassium, thiamin, and riboflavin.

Baking soda: Cleanser, soother, and softener used in scrubs and masques; softens water; also known as bicarbonate of soda; high alkaline levels give it gentle (nonacidic) cleansing power.

Banana (plantain): Humectant and moisturizer used in facial and body masques, scrubs, and baths; produced by a herbaceous plant; high in potassium and vitamin C.

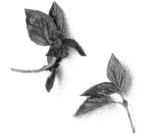

Basil: Hair growth stimulant, hair conditioner, and detangler; skin soother and stimulant; member of the mint family with strong licorice flavor; main ingredient in pesto sauce.

Bay laurel: Aromatic, antiseptic, stimulant, and soother; reduces swelling and inflammation in joints; native to the Mediterranean.

Beer: Skin conditioner and soother; hair volumizer; alcoholic beverage brewed primarily from malted barley, yeast, hops, and water.

Binder: Increases consistency of products; holds ingredients together in a masque, peel, or scrub to increase their adhesion to the skin or hair; eggs, gelatin, and pectin are commonly used as binders in recipes.

Black tea: Soother, astringent, anti-inflammatory, sunburn treatment; native to China; leaves from tea plant have been fermented for intensity and strength.

Bok choy: Toner, astringent, and soother; also known as Chinese white cabbage with mild, crunchy stalks.

Broccoli: Moisturizer with vitamins A and C, riboflavin, calcium, and iron; related to cabbage.

Brown rice: Soother of irritated skin, conditioner; ancient grain grown in flooded plains or tropical terrain; high in fiber, B vitamins, vitamin E, calcium, and iron; available in supermarkets or health food stores.

Brussels sprouts: Moisturizer in hair and facial masques; contains vitamins A, C, and small amounts of D and some iron; from the cabbage family; grown in fall and winter.

Buttermilk: Mild exfoliant; emollient and skin conditioner; gives skin a rosy flow; fermented dairy product that contains lactic acid, said to stimulate cell growth.

Calendula: Healant, soother, hair lightener; flower is also called pot marigold; available loose in health food stores.

Canola oil: Occlusive oil; emollient; also known as "rapeseed oil"; polyunsaturated fat.

Cantaloupe: Soother and refresher with vitamins A and C; good for dry skin; also called muskmelon or rock melon; rough, tan exterior with sweet orange flesh; summer fruit; member of the squash family.

Carrot: Soother, antiseptic, cleanser, contains beta carotene, precursor of vitamin A.

Castor oil: Occlusive oil; emollient used in moisturizers and nail creams; used to remove makeup; from the pressed beans of the castor plant.

Celery: Astringent, toner, tonic for skin; member of the carrot family long used as a medicinal herb.

Chamomile: Soother, healant, anti-inflammatory, diaphoretic, refresher, pore cleanser; lightens blonde hair; aromatic flower often used in soothing teas; available sold as tea loose or in bags in supermarkets or health food stores.

Cherimoya: Soothing skin conditioner; moisturizer; used in facial and body masques and scrubs; tough, green exterior with creamy, custardlike interior with black seeds; tropical fruit available in winter and early spring.

Cilantro (coriander leaves): Aromatic, stimulant; Mediterranean and Asian herb related to parsley; available fresh only.

Cinnamon: Stimulant and bactericide; anti-inflammatory; used ground as a dark hair rinse and hair scent; ancient spice from inner bark of a tropical evergreen tree; sweet, savory flavor.

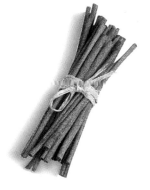

Citric acid: Oil remover or reducer; found primarily in citrus fruits, such as lemons; used in toners, facial masques, scrubs, and oil-reducing shampoos and hair rinses.

Cleanser: A substance that loosens particles of grime and facilitates the removal of dirt and oils.

Clove: Astringent, antiseptic, aromatic, stimulant; spice from flower bud grown on tropical evergreen clove tree; named from Latin "clavus" meaning nail (shaped); available whole or ground.

Coconut milk: Cleansing emollient; skin smoother; made from grated coconut meat and water heated together and pressed; available canned.

Coconut oil: Emollient, moisturizer, scent; opaque saturated fat made by pressing coconut meat.

Coffee: Soothing anti-inflammatory; dark hair rinse; roasted beans from coffee plant.

Collard greens: Softener and skin conditioner used in masques and scrubs; contain vitamins A and C and iron; leafy, dark green vegetable.

Corn (yellow): Starchy toner, astringent; contains vitamin A; kernel from fruit of corn plant.

Cornmeal: Exfoliant used in masques and scrubs; from ground corn kernels.

Corn oil: Occlusive oil; emollient; from the endosperm of corn kernels; polyunsaturated oil.

Cornstarch (corn flour): Body powder; absorbs odor and wetness; floury substance from endosperm of corn kernel; used as thickening agent.

Couscous: Exfoliant used in scrubs and masques; granular semolina, classified as pasta, used in North African cuisine; available in supermarkets or specialty food stores.

Cucumber: Astringent and toner; mild exfoliant with bleaching action; healant for irritated, sunburned, wrinkled, or hardened skin; from the squash family.

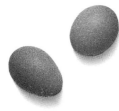

Egg: Skin conditioner and toner; helps reduce appearance of pores on skin; hair volumizer and thickener; used to bind other ingredients together.

Emollient: A skin-conditioning agent that helps to keep the soft and smooth appearance of the skin; acts as a lubricant and leaves a silky finish on the skin's surface or in the first layer of skin.

Exfoliant: An ingredient that sheds the superficial, dead skin cells; peels skin away using acids, enzymes, or abrasion. Removal of dead skin cells encourages new cell growth and improves appearance of skin.

Extract: Emollient and skin conditioner; scent; concentration from a food substance, through evaporation or mixing with a solvent, such as water.

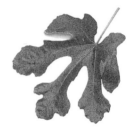

Fig: Skin cleanser and soother; anti-inflammatory; mild exfoliant used in scrubs and creams; Mediterranean fruit with soft flesh containing tiny seeds; skin ranges from dark purple to pale cream; extremely perishable; should be used immediately; available fresh from June to late October; contains iron, calcium, and phosphorus.

Garbanzo beans (chickpeas): Skin moisturizer and conditioner used in body masques; a tan-colored legume used in Mediterranean and Asian cooking; main ingredient in hummus; found canned or dry.

Gelatin: Thickens and gelatinizes recipes; used in body and facial masques; derived from livestock bones, cartilage, and tissue. Vegetarian alternative is pectin.

Ginger: Antiseptic for skin; stimulant; root from tropical plant; knobby, coarse exterior with stringy, pungent, peppery flesh; available dried or fresh; used to flavor foods, drinks, and confections; caution should be used with ginger; may cause skin irritation.

Grape: Soothing anti-inflammatory; exfoliant; skin softener; grows in clusters on shrubs or vines; contains small amounts of vitamins A and C and enzymes.

Grapefruit: Exfoliant and cleanser; oil remover; member of the citrus family; contains citric acid and vitamin C.

Hair conditioner: An ingredient that enhances the appearance of the hair, improving shine, body, and texture.

Hazelnut oil: Moisturizer, scent, and emollient for skin; pressed from hazelnuts; turns rancid quickly, so store in refrigerator.

Healant: Healing agent for irritated or chapped skin; a medicine that heals skin abrasions or skin conditions such as psoriasis.

Hearts of palm: Skin conditioner and emollient used in masques and scrubs; fleshy interior of cabbage palm tree stem; grown in tropical climate; fresh is difficult to obtain; sold primarily in cans

Honey: Humectant; skin conditioner and emollient; gentle cleanser; used in moisturizers, scrubs, masques, and cleansers; made by bees using flower nectar; flavor and color varies based on the flower from which the nectar is drawn.

Honeydew melon: Soother and refresher with vitamin C; good for dry skin; used in facial masques and scrubs; smooth, pale yellow or green exterior with similarly colored, sweet flesh; summer fruit; member of the squash family.

Humectant: Used in cosmetics to slow down or stop loss of moisture from the skin; increases water content in the first layer of skin.

Hydrogen peroxide: Germicide and antiseptic; cleanser and anti-inflammatory used in toners and facial sprays; chemical formula is H_2O_2. Don't use on broken skin.

Iceberg lettuce: Soother, refresher, and astringent used in facial and body toner; variety of crisphead lettuce; crisp and succulent leaves.

Kale: Skin softener and nutrient used in scrubs; contains vitamins A and C, folic acid, calcium, and iron; from the cabbage family; rich, dark green leaves with varying shades of color, including purple and blue.

Kidney bean: Skin conditioner and softener used in scrubs and masques; a dark red legume with cream-colored interior; high in protein, iron, and B vitamins.

Kiwi: Soother, refresher, and skin conditioner used in masques and toners; contains vitamin C; also known as Chinese gooseberry; tropical fruit with rough brown skin and bright green, tangy flesh containing small black seeds.

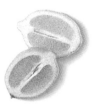

Lemon: Astringent, toner, exfoliant, and oil remover used in scrubs, toners, masques, and hair rinses; hair lightener; member of the citrus family containing vitamin C; oil is from pressing of rind.

Lemongrass: Astringent; refresher; cleanser and oil regulator used in cleansers and scrubs; resembles a green onion or scallion, with bitter lemony taste and smell; flavors many Southeast Asian dishes.

Lima bean: Skin conditioner and softener; a plump, pale green legume with protein, potassium, and iron; named for birthplace, Lima, Peru. A staple in Africa, also known as Madagascar bean.

Lime: Astringent, refresher, exfoliant, and oil remover used in toners and scrubs; hair lightener; dark green-skinned member of the citrus family with soft, pale green flesh; contains vitamin C.

Long-grain rice: Soother of irritated skin, toner and skin conditioner used in scrubs and masques; variety of ancient grain grown in flooded plain or tropical terrain; high in fiber, B vitamins, calcium, and iron.

Macadamia nut oil: Moisturizing emollient used in body and facial moisturizers; high in fat, with 80 calories per nut. Native to Australia, grows on an evergreen tree; largest producer is Hawaii.

Mango: Skin softener and conditioner used in masques and scrubs; contains vitamins A, C, and small amounts of D. Lush, tropical fruit with orange flesh encased in tough skin that turns creamy red when ripened.

Maple syrup: Humectant, softener, and conditioner used in facial masques and scrubs and hair shampoos. Derived from boiling the sap of the maple tree.

Mayonnaise: Softener and emollient; occlusive skin conditioner. Emulsion of egg yolk, vegetable oil, and lemon or vinegar; high in fat.

Milk: Soothing moisturizer; skin softener and emollient; cleanser; skin lightener; whole, lowfat, nonfat, and skim varieties contain varying amounts of butterfat; contains vitamins A and D.

Millet: Exfoliant used in scrubs and masques. A cereal grain from the grass family, it is rich in protein; food staple for much of the world; used in the United States primarily as fodder and bird seed; very small grains. Found in health food stores.

Mint: Stimulant, invigorator, and scent used in baths, masques, scrubs, and cleansers; creates a cold stimulus that triggers the brain to create warming trends in affected areas of skin. Fragrant, bright green leaves; best when used fresh. Oil is highly concentrated and has drying effect.

Moisturizer: An emollient, which makes skin feel softer and smoother; reduces roughness, cracking, and irritation of the skin.

Mustard greens: Stimulant, anti-inflammatory, and pain reliever used in soaks and baths; member of the cabbage family; has a tart, peppery flavor. Leaves range from deep green to shades of yellow red. Dried form is from ground mustard seeds.

Napa cabbage: Toner, soother, and astringent with vitamin A, folic acid, and potassium; also called Chinese cabbage; crinkly, delicate leaves.

Oats (quick rolled): Soother, skin softener, and cleanser; mild exfoliant used in scrubs, cleansers, masques, baths, and sunburn treatments; a cereal grass with substantial fat content, B vitamins and vitamin E, rolled oats are made from toasted, hulled oat grains.

Occlusive oil: An oil that increases the water content of the skin by creating a seal on the surface, holding in moisture.

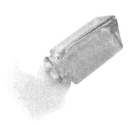

Olive oil: Softening, occlusive emollient used in moisturizers, masques, and scrubs; made by pressing olives; a monounsaturated oil; olives grow in mild climates, primarily around the Mediterranean.

Orange oil: A scented emollient; skin softener used in moisturizers and scrubs; extracted by pressing the orange rind.

Oregano: Hair detangler and softener; rinse for dark hair. Member of the mint family, a pungent, strong herb that is used in Mediterranean and Mexican cooking.

Papaya (paw paw): Exfoliant and skin conditioner used in scrubs and masques; tropical fruit that contains golden fruit with black seeds. Contains vitamins A and C and a protein-digesting enzyme, papain.

Parsley: Healant, cleanser, soother used for psoriasis, eczema, acne, and blemishes; contains vitamins A and C. A member of the carrot family, this ubiquitous herb is often used to garnish and flavor foods.

Peach: Soother, softener, and skin conditioner used in facial and body masques and scrubs; contains vitamins A and C. A member of the rose family, this summer fruit has tender, orange flesh encased in a soft, rosy skin; native to China.

Peanut oil: Occlusive oil; emollient for skin used in moisturizers and masques; polyunsaturated oil; pressed from peanuts.

Pear: Soother and skin conditioner; anti-inflammatory used in masques and scrubs. A member of the rose family, it has pale yellow flesh with a variety of skin colors and textures.

Peas: Moisturizer and skin conditioner used in masques and scrubs; contains vitamins A and C. A bright green legume, it originated in the Middle East.

Pectin: Binder and thickener used in scrubs, gels, and masques to hold ingredients together in order to adhere more easily to the skin; a natural thickener found in fruits and vegetables. Vegetarian alternative to gelatin.

Pineapple: Exfoliant, soother, anti-inflammatory, and refresher used in facial and body masques and scrubs; contains bromelin, a protein-digesting enzyme. Tropical fruit that grows on a low bush, contains vitamins A and C.

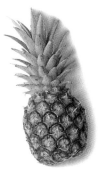

Pine nuts (pignoli): Skin softener and conditioner used in masques and scrubs; high-fat nut that grows on pine or "pignon" trees and is found inside the pine cone. Smooth, creamy white color and texture; main ingredient in pesto; becomes rancid easily, so refrigerate. Found in health food stores.

Powdered milk: Soother and softener; skin conditioner used in masques, scrubs, and cleansers. Dehydrated milk, available in whole, lowfat, and nonfat varieties; fortified with vitamins A and C.

Pumpkin: Moisturizer; emollient; skin conditioner and smoother used in body masques and moisturizers and hair packs; contains vitamin A. A member of the squash family, it has a hard, round, orange body with bright orange flesh and large, flat seeds.

Quinoa: Exfoliant used in scrubs and masques; high in protein, it contains all essential amino acids, as well as vitamin E and a number of B vitamins. An ancient grain used by the Incas in Peru, it is a great source of nutrients. Subtle, grainy flavor in small, round, granular shape. Found in supermarkets and health food stores.

Refried beans: Moisturizer and skin and hair conditioner used in masques and packs; high in protein. Made from mash of beans and lard. Vegetarian variety uses vegetable shortening or oil. Staple in Mexican cuisine.

Rice bran oil: Occlusive emollient and skin conditioner; derived from the outer layer of rice.

Rosemary: Stimulant and astringent; darkens and conditions hair; used in shampoos, hair rinses, and body scrubs and masques. Fragrant member of the mint family; native to the Mediterranean.

Rum: Oil reducer and remover used in shampoos and facial toners. Derived from distillation of fermented sugar cane juice or molasses, produced primarily in the Caribbean. Available as white or silver as well as a golden, amber variety.

Russet potato: Astringent, toner, mild exfoliant, skin lightener, and healant used in toners, masques, cleansers, and scrubs; contains potassium and vitamin C. Ancient tuber cultivated in Peru; thousands of varieties grown. Russet has brown, rough skin and dense, pale cream flesh.

Sage: Antiseptic and soother; stimulant and hair darkener used in hair rinses and body and facial masques and scrubs. A member of the mint family, it is an ancient medicinal herb, used to accent meats and vegetables.

Salt: Soother; blister medicant used in sunburn treatments and facial masques. Extracted from salt mines or from the sea.

Sesame oil: Occlusive emollient used in moisturizers and masques; fragrant, polyunsaturated oil extracted from pressing sesame seeds.

Sesame seeds: Exfoliant and moisturizing emollient used in body and facial scrubs and masques. Ancient seed with high oil content; turns rancid quickly so keep refrigerated.

Shampoo: Where the recipes in this book call for shampoo in the ingredients list, any shampoo product can be used. However, do note the recipes which specify *not* to use certain types of products, such as one-step (with conditioners) or dandruff shampoo.

Shortening: Occlusive emollient used in moisturizers, masques, and scrubs; hydrogenated vegetable oil, primarily from soybean and cottonseed oils.

Skin conditioner: An emollient, humectant, or occlusive agent found in foods.

Smoother: An ingredient that gives a smooth, more even texture to the skin.

Solvent: A liquid that dissolves ingredients used in cosmetics.

Soother: An ingredient that relieves pain or stinging on the flesh.

Soybean: High in fat; softens and conditions the skin.

Spaghetti squash: Moisturizing emollient used in masques and scrubs; contains vitamins A and C and iron; large, hard yellow shell filled with tender, yellow flesh.

Spinach: Soother, nutrient, and skin conditioner used in masques and scrubs; contains vitamins A and C. Dark green, crisp leafy vegetable available year round.

Stimulant: A chemical that increases circulation and excites the senses.

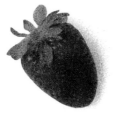

Strawberry: Astringent, cleanser, and skin conditioner used in scrubs and masques; contains vitamin C, iron, and potassium. Juicy, red fruit; member of the rose family.

Strawberry papaya: Exfoliant and skin conditioner used in scrubs and masques; a variety of regular papaya, a tropical fruit; flesh is pinkish, resembling strawberries, and contains black seeds. Contains vitamins A and C and a protein-digesting enzyme, papain.

Sweet potato: Moisturizer, emollient, nutrient, and skin conditioner used in body masques and scrubs; contains vitamins A and C. Native of Central America, this large root has a skin ranging from pale yellow to deep brown-orange with yellow to orange flesh inside.

Tarragon: Stimulant used in body masques and hair rinses; fragrant herb native to Asia; important component in béarnaise sauce.

Thyme: Aromatic, antiseptic stimulant; diaphoretic used in facial masques and toners and rinses for hair. A fragrant member of the mint family, this herb has been used since ancient times for medicinal purposes.

Tightener: An ingredient that leaves a toned, tightened sensation on the skin.

Toner: A substance that tightens the skin; an astringent; temporarily closes pores; improves textures of skin.

Vitamin A: Contained in its precursor, beta carotene, found in yellow and green vegetables; helps heal the epithelia cells, that is, the epidermis or top layer of skin; may pass through the skin's layers, creating a healthier appearance.

Vitamin B: Found in fruits, vegetables, and grains; some evidence exists that B6 is a skin-conditioning agent. B1 and B2 are occlusive skin conditioners, but never pass through the epidermis.

Vitamin C: Found in numerous fruits and vegetables; can pass through the layers of the skin and is a healant for abrasions and burns.

Vitamin D: Found in fruits, vegetables, dairy products, and the sun; has a healing effect on the skin; is absorbed through the layers of the skin.

Vodka: Astringent and oil remover used in facial toners and cleansers and oil-reducing shampoos and rinses. An alcoholic beverage from distilled potatoes or grains.

Walnut oil: Occlusive emollient used in moisturizers and skin conditioners; pressed from the walnut; high fat content that increases rancidity, so keep refrigerated.

Water chestnut: Exfoliant, moisturizer; indigenous to Southeast Asia.

Watercress: Astringent; medicant; member of the mustard family.

Watermelon: Astringent and skin conditioner used in facial masques; especially good for oily skin. Contains small amounts of vitamins A and C. A member of the squash family, this summer fruit has a hard green or green and white shell containing bright red or yellow flesh, speckled with black seeds. Seedless varieties exist, but are more expensive.

Wheat germ: Soother, emollient, skin conditioner used in scrubs and masques; contains vitamin E. Extracted from the wheat grain, it is the embryo of the berry, with a high fat content, increasing rancidity, so keep refrigerated.

Whipping cream: Soothing moisturizer, skin softener, and emollient; binder; has a high butterfat content; produced by separating unhomogenized milk.

White mushroom: Skin conditioner and emollient used in scrubs and cleansers; contains potassium and B vitamins; edible fungus; clean with dry, soft cloth; do not wash off.

White vinegar (distilled): Astringent and oil remover used in facial toners and scrubs; made from fermented grain alcohol.

White wine: Astringent and oil remover used in facial toners; fermented juice of white grapes or the flesh but not the skin of red grape varietals. Wine has been produced for thousands of years. Dry white wines are best for toners.

Witch hazel: Astringent, antiseptic, healant, oil remover used in scrubs, toners, and masques. An aromatic extract from low-lying shrub, it is gentle enough for all skin types.

Yogurt: Emollient; skin conditioner; mild exfoliant and cleanser; gives skin a rosy flow; fermented milk product with tangy taste; available in regular, low-fat, and nonfat; contains lactic acid, said to stimulate cell growth.

Bibliography

The Aphrodisiac Gourmet, Eric Hill, Aries Publishing, Hayward, CA, 1982.

Basic Food Chemistry, Frank A. Lee, Ph.D., The AVI Publishing Co., Inc., Westport, CT, 1975.

Beauty Is Skin Deep, Howard Donasky, M.D., Rodale Press, Emmaus, Pennsylvania, 1985.

Bullfinch's Complete Mythology, Spring Books, London, 1989.

Chilies to Chocolate: Food the Americas Gave the World, ed. Nelson Foster & Linda S. Cordell, The University of Arizona Press, Tucson & London, 1992.

The Complete Book of Beans, Jacqueline Heriteau, Hawthorn Books, Inc., New York, 1978.

A Consumer's Dictionary of Cosmetic Ingredients, Ruth Winter, Crown Publishers, Inc., New York, 1989, 3rd ed.

Craig Claiborne's The New York Times Food Encyclopedia, Craig Claiborne, Wings Books, New York, 1994.

Don't Swallow the Avocado Pit—and What to Do with the Rest of It, Helen Rosenbaum, Paul S. Eriksson, Inc., New York, 1974.

Down to Earth Beauty, Catherine Palmer, St. Martin's Press, New York, 1981.

The Essential Root Vegetable Cookbook, Sally and Martin Stone, Clarkson Potter, New York, 1991.

Food and Culture in America, Pamela Goyan Kittler and Kathryn Sucher, Van Nostrand Reinhold, New York, 1989.

The Food Factor: Why We Are What We Eat, Barbara Griggs, Viking Press, New York 1986.

Food Lover's Companion, Sharon Tyler Herbst, Barron's, Hauppauge, NY, 1990.

The Grains Book, Bert Greene, Workman Publishing, New York, 1988.

The Great Food Almanac: A Feast of Facts from A to Z, Irena Chalmers, Collin Publishers, San Francisco, 1994.

The Healing Foods Cookbook, ed. Jean Rogers (from editors of *Prevention Magazine*), Rodale Press, Emmaus, PA, 1991.

Health Foods & Herbs, Kathleen Hunter, ARC Books, Inc., New York, 1963.

Herb Identifier and Handbook, Ingrid Gabriel, Sterling Publishing Co., Inc., New York, 1979.

The Herbal Body Book: A Natural Approach to Healthier Hair, Skin and Nails, Stephanie L. Tourles, Storey Communications, Inc., Pownal, VT, 1994.

History of Food, Maguelonne Toussaint-Samat, trans. by Anthea Bell, Blackwell Publishers, Cambridge, MA, 1992.

Jane Grigson's Fruit Book, Jane Grigson, Atheneum, New York, 1982.

Jeanne Rose's Herbal Body Book, Jeanne Rose, ill. by Michael S. Moore, Grosset & Dunlap, New York, 1976.

Kitchen Wisdom, Pamela Cross, Camden House, Columbia, SC, 1991.

Lia Schorr's Seasonal Skin Care, Lia Schorr with Shari Miller Sims, Prentice Hall Press, New York, 1988.

Liz Earle's Natural Beauty, Liz Earle, Vermilion, London, 1993.

A Modern Herbal, Volumes I and II, Mrs. M. Grieve, Dover Publications, Inc., New York, 1982.

Natural Health and Beauty, Bronwen Meredith, Holt, Rinehart and Winston, New York, 1979.

Natural Skin Care, Sherie de Haas, Avery Publishing Group, Inc., Garden City Park, NY, 1987.

The New Medically Based No-Nonsense Beauty Book, Deborah Chase, ill. by Margaret Garrison, Henry Holt & Co., New York, 1989.

On Food and Cooking: The Science and Lore of the Kitchen, Harold McGee, Collier Books, MacMillan Publishing, New York, 1984.

The Secret Life of Food, Martin Elkort, Jeremy P. Tarcher, Los Angeles, 1991.

Index

Chamomile, 39, 87

*Chamomile and Calendula Hair
Lightener*, 87

*Chamomile-Fig Eye and Facial
Soother*, 65

Chamomile tea, 61, 65

Cherimoya, 37

*Cherimoya-Couscous Moisturizing
Facial Scrub*, 37

Cherry-Almond Hair Mist, 88

Cherry-Almond Shampoo Additive, 92

Cherry extract, 88, 92

Chocolate extract, 91

*Chocolate-Pumpkin Conditioning Hair
Milk*, 91, 124

Cilantro, 18

Cinnamon extract, 101

Cinnamon oil, 100, 101, 107

*Cinnamon-Pineapple Foot Rub with
Mint*, 107

Citrus Hair Lightener, 90

Clove and Apple Dandruff Shampoo, 83

Cloves, 83

Coconut extract, 13, 17, 21, 27, 38,
49, 103

Coconut milk, 6, 25, 50, 78, 80, 81,
91, 102

Coconut oil, 5, 12, 14, 19, 26, 34, 38, 50,
76, 80, 91, 93, 103, 110

Coconut Tanning Oil, 110

Coco Palm Facial Moisturizer, 38

Collard greens, 16

Conversion chart, 125

Cooling Psoriasis Relief Treatment, 108

Corn, 10

Corn oil, 12, 13

Cornstarch, 27

Couscous, 37

Cream, 6, 8, 17, 39, 40

Creamy Cucumber Facial Cleanser,
32, 120

Cucumber extract, xiii, 4, 10, 12, 17, 109

Cucumber-Parsley Facial Toner, 46, 122

Cucumbers, 6, 9, 21, 24, 32, 39, 40, 47,
49, 54, 58, 59, 61, 65, 98, 102, 111,
114, 116

E

Eggs
  whites, 9, 10, 17, 21, 32, 33, 42, 44,
    50, 53, 54, 55, 57, 59, 61, 62
  whole, 8, 25, 32, 40, 41, 44, 73, 74,
    80, 82, 92, 106
  yolks, 84, 105

Equatorial Enzyme Pack, 9, 121

Extracts, xii
  almond, 4, 9, 11, 13, 14, 20, 35, 39,
    47, 49, 50, 54, 55, 88, 91, 92, 117
  anise, 37, 100, 106, 113
  banana, 6, 17, 25, 34, 50, 82
  cherry, 88, 92
  chocolate, 91
  cinnamon, 101
  coconut, 13, 17, 21, 27, 38, 49, 103
  cucumber, xiii, 4, 10, 12, 17, 109
  lemon, 6, 24, 34, 39, 41, 47, 55, 67,
    72, 74, 75, 82, 84, 87, 89, 90, 98,
    103, 106, 109, 116
  lime, 34, 41, 45, 47, 90, 103
  maple, 6
  orange, 11, 27, 34, 49, 67, 75, 82, 101
  peppermint, 20, 73, 98, 99, 107
  pineapple, 39
  rum, 72, 83
  vanilla, 21, 34, 74, 85, 88, 91, 92

F

Facial care
  all skin types, 32, 35, 37, 40, 44, 45,
    48, 52–55, 58, 60, 61, 62, 64, 65
  mature skin, 33, 38
  nonsensitive skin, 35
  normal to dry skin, 35, 41, 46, 49, 50
  oily skin, 35, 47, 59, 66

Strawberry papaya, 53, 67
Summer, specific recipes for, 121–22
Sun Blister Skin Treatment, 115
Suntanning Soothing and Cleansing Mist, 109
Syrup, maple, 92

T

Tarragon, 106
Tea
    black, 11, 20, 22, 45, 53, 65, 89, 108, 111, 114, 115
    chamomile, 61, 65
    oolong, 116
Tests, patch, xiii
Three-Bean Body Salad Skin-Conditioning Body Masque, 16
Thyme, 20, 48, 52
Tropical Facial Frappé, 35

V

Vanilla extract, 21, 34, 74, 85, 88, 91, 92
Vanilla-Rum Cocktail, 74, 122
Vegetable oil, 8, 38, 91, 110
Vegetable shortening, 5, 16, 38, 52, 93
Vegetarian Refried Bean Hair Masque, 78, 123
Vinegar
    apple cider, 6, 27, 46, 75, 77, 83, 84, 105
    white, 116
Vodka, 49, 75

W

Walnut oil, 19
Water chestnuts, 37
Watercress, 27, 37, 57, 58, 59, 60, 62, 66, 67, 113
Watercress and Rice Acne Facial Toner, 66
Watercress-Papaya Acne Cleanser, 67
Watermelon, 18
Wheat germ, 21, 24, 50, 106
Wheat germ oil, 103
Whipped Oatmeal-Sesame Seed Scrub Cream, 39
White Wine and Mint Blemish Treatment Masque, 58
Wine, white, 58
Winter, specific recipes for, 123–24
Witch hazel, 48, 49
Witch Hazel-Vodka Conditioning Facial Toners, 49

Y

Yogurt, 11, 32, 37, 40, 42, 44, 55
    nonfat, 32, 40, 44, 55